# POINT-OF-CARE ULTRASOUND POCKET GUIDE

**Kelli Craven, DNP, ENP-C, AGACNP-BC, FNP-BC, NRP,** has worked in emergency medicine for over 25 years. She is multi–board certified with a focus on emergency medicine and critical care in rural health. Currently, Dr. Craven functions in multiple locum assignments at various trauma-designated hospitals and critical access facilities. She is a course developer for educational content focused on ultrasound skills development within the learning management system and national conferences with the American Academy of Emergency Nurse Practitioners (AAENP). She is active in various leadership roles for the AAENP as a state representative for Arizona and South Dakota and serves as an educational committee member. She has also functioned in the chief hospitalist role for critical access hospitals. She maintains active certifications and her national registered paramedic license to continue working in the pre-hospital environment. She has presented her doctoral work at national conferences and has guest lectured for Arizona State University's ENP program and precepted ENP students from both Arizona State University and Vanderbilt University School of Nursing.

**Wesley Davis, DNP, ENP-C, FNP-C, AGACNP-BC, PMHNP-C, CEN, FAANP, FAEN, FAAN,** is an Associate Professor and Dual Family/Emergency Nurse Practitioner Program Director at the University of South Alabama College of Nursing. With more than 25 years of experience as an emergency nurse across diverse clinical settings, Dr. Davis is a nationally recognized leader in emergency and trauma nursing and has been extensively published in the field. Dr. Davis is a past president of the American Academy of Emergency Nurse Practitioners (AAENP) and currently serves as Associate Editor of the Advanced Emergency Nursing Journal. He also led the 2021 revision of the Emergency Nurse Practitioner (ENP) competencies, a collaborative initiative between AAENP and the Emergency Nurses Association that helped strengthen national standards for emergency nurse practitioner education and practice. He is the author of the *Emergency Nurse Practitioner Scope and Standards*, co-published by Springer Publishing and AAENP in 2023, which serves as a foundational resource for emergency nurse practitioner practice and education. In addition, Dr. Davis chairs the AAENP Validation Program, which establishes national standards for academic emergency nurse practitioner programs to promote educational rigor, quality, and integrity. He also leads national initiatives advancing the emergency nurse practitioner specialty toward formal recognition as an APRN population focus, helping shape the future of emergency advanced practice nursing education and regulation in the United States. In clinical practice, Dr. Davis serves as Chief of Staff for the Crook County Medical Services District and as County Health Officer for Crook County Public Health in Sundance, Wyoming.

# POINT-OF-CARE ULTRASOUND POCKET GUIDE

*Kelli Craven, DNP, ENP-C, AGACNP-BC, FNP-BC, NRP*
Lead Editor


*Wesley Davis, DNP, ENP-C, FNP-C, AGACNP-BC, PMHNP-C, CEN, FAANP, FAEN, FAAN*
Editor

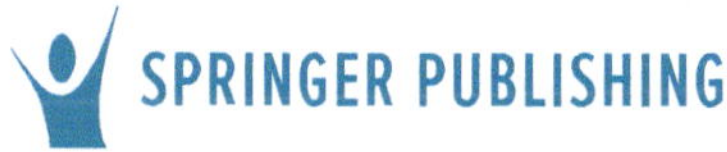

Springer Publishing Company, LLC
902 Carnegie Center, Princeton, NJ 08540
www.springerpub.com
connect.springerpub.com

*Acquisitions Editor*: John Zaphyr
*Compositor*: S4Carlisle Publishing Services
*Production Editor*: Kris Parrish

*ISBN*: 978-0-8261-3854-5
*e-book ISBN*: 978-0-8261-3855-2
*DOI*: 10.1891/9780826138552

26 27 28 29 / 5 4 3 2 1

Medicine is an ever-changing science. Research and clinical experience are continually expanding our knowledge, in particular our understanding of proper treatment and drug therapy. The authors, editors, and publisher have made every effort to ensure that all information in this book is in accordance with the state of knowledge at the time of production of the book. Nevertheless, the authors, editors, and publisher are not responsible for any errors or omissions or for any consequence from application of the information in this book and make no warranty, expressed or implied, with respect to the content of this publication. Every reader should examine carefully the package inserts accompanying each drug and should carefully check whether the dosage schedules therein or the contraindications stated by the manufacturer differ from the statements made in this book. Such examination is particularly important with drugs that are either rarely used or have been newly released on the market.



**Library of Congress Control Number: 2025026319**

Contact sales@springerpub.com to receive discount rates on bulk purchases.

*Publisher's Note:* **New and used products purchased from third-party sellers are not guaranteed for quality, authenticity, or access to any included digital components.**

Printed in the United States of America by Gasch Printing.

*This book is dedicated to all my friends and family who have supported my journey to make a difference in healthcare and to all those in the field of medicine who sacrifice their lives every day in efforts to improve patient outcomes.*

*To God be the glory!*

# CONTENTS

# CONTRIBUTORS

**Marlen Alvarez, DNP, FNP-C, ENP-C**
Emergency Nurse Practitioner Fellow
UT Southwestern Medical Center
Dalton, Georgia

**John Barrett, DNP**
Nurse Practitioner
Penn Medicine
Philadelphia, Pennsylvania

**Ari Chaskes, DNP, FNP-BC, ENP-C**
Emergency Nurse Practitioner
Sound Physicians
Frederick, Maryland

**Kelli Craven, DNP, ENP-C, AGACNP-BC, FNP-BC, NRP**
Board-Certified Nurse Practitioner
Paradigm Health, PLLC CEO
AAENP State Representative & US Committee Chair
Wanblee, South Dakota

**Wesley Davis, DNP, ENP-C, FNP-C, AGACNP-BC, PMHNP-C, CEN, FAANP, FAEN, FAAN**
Associate Professor
Dual Family/Emergency Nurse Practitioner Program Director
University of South Alabama College of Nursing
Mobile, Alabama

**Adriana De La Rue, PA-C**
Emergency Medicine Physician Assistant
UT Southwestern Medical Center
Carrollton, Texas

**Christopher Deonarine, MPAS, PA-C**
Anesthesiology and Pain Management
UT Southwestern Medical Center
Dalton, Georgia

**Juan M. Gonzalez, DNP, APRN, AGACNP-BC, ENP-C, FNP-BC, CEN, CNE, FAANP**
Associate Professor of Clinical, Adult Gerontology Acute Care Program Director
University of Miami School of Nursing and Health Studies
Miami, Florida

**Meghan Petzy, MSN, FNP, ENP**
Emergency Nurse Practitioner
Mass General Brigham—Wentworth Douglass Hospital
Portsmouth, New Hampshire

# PREFACE

Point-of-care ultrasound (POCUS) is the future of medicine at the bedside and in the pre-hospital environment. With the shortage of medical professionals at various levels, it is critical the medical team begin to think outside the box regarding how we can improve patient outcomes. POCUS is the answer to overcoming identified barriers with staffing shortages, high volumes, overrun emergency departments, low resources, and increasingly complex medical diagnoses. Fast-paced critical care environments have minimal time to develop care plans, meet benchmarks, and maintain standards of care. The use of POCUS has largely become the standard of care for procedural guidance and exceeds benchmarks reducing door to diagnosis, door to pain management, door to treatment, door to discharge, and complications during invasive procedures. This publication seeks to solve the time constraints in learning POCUS at the bedside. *The Point-of Care Ultrasound Pocket Guide* is a quick reference for the diagnostic and procedural scans most commonly encountered in any setting both in and outside the hospital. This guide allows those who have had formal or informal POCUS training to embark on a journey to improve their skills and competency and empowers all providers at the bedside. Readers can learn POCUS and obtain real-time images improving patient care outcomes using non-ionizing radiation. QR codes within certain chapters provide live scan images demonstrating proper transducer placement, patient position, and scanner position for obtaining quality images. Learn it, love it, and always scan it!

# ACKNOWLEDGMENTS

We like to personally acknowledge all the contributors and authors for their dedication and commitment to the success of the publication. A special thank you to Dr. Ari Chaskes and Mrs. Meg Petzy for their unwavering collaboration on video production.

# LIST OF VIDEOS

Airway
*Chapter 23, Surgical Airway*

Arthrocentesis
*Chapter 17, Paracentesis, Pericardiocentesis, Arthrocentesis, Thoracentesis*

Cardiac Introduction
*Chapter 6, Point-of-Care Ultrasound Cardiac Echocardiography*

Estimating Ejection Fraction
*Chapter 6, Point-of-Care Ultrasound Cardiac Echocardiography*

Extended Focused Assessment With Sonography in Trauma (E-FAST) Exam
*Chapter 4, Extended Focus Assessment With Sonography in Trauma (E-FAST Exam)*

## Pericardial Effusion
*Chapter 6, Point-of-Care Ultrasound Cardiac Echocardiography;*
*Chapter 17, Paracentesis, Pericardiocentesis, Arthrocentesis,*
*Thoracentesis*

## Pericardiocentesis
*Chapter 17, Paracentesis, Pericardiocentesis, Arthrocentesis,*
*Thoracentesis*

## Pleural Effusion—Thoracentesis
*Chapter 10, Lung Ultrasound Exam; Chapter 17, Paracentesis,*
*Pericardiocentesis, Arthrocentesis, Thoracentesis*

## Pleural Evaluation in Extended Focused Assessment With Sonography in Trauma (E-FAST) Exam
*Chapter 4, Extended Focus Assessment With*
*Sonography in Trauma (E-FAST Exam); Chapter 10,*
*Lung Ultrasound Exam*

## Renal Ultrasound
*Chapter 8, Renal Ultrasound*

## Right Ventricle Function
*Chapter 6, Point-of-Care Ultrasound Cardiac Echocardiography*

## Subxiphoid/Subcostal View
*Chapter 4, Extended Focus Assessment With Sonography in Trauma (E-FAST Exam); Chapter 6, Point-of-Care Ultrasound Cardiac Echocardiography; Chapter 17, Paracentesis, Pericardiocentesis, Arthrocentesis, Thoracentesis*

## Thoracentesis
*Chapter 17, Paracentesis, Pericardiocentesis, Arthrocentesis, Thoracentesis*

## Transabdominal View
*Chapter 13, First Trimester Pregnancy*

# CHAPTER 1

# INTRODUCTION TO POINT-OF-CARE ULTRASOUND

Marlen Alvarez and Kelli Craven

## EVOLUTION OF ULTRASOUND

- **1950s:** immersion tanks produced first 2-D images
- **1960s–1970s:** use in obstetrics catapulted ultrasound development
- **1965:** first US machine produced
- **1980s:** use of ultrasound in emergency medicine
- **1990s:** introduction of point-of-care ultrasound (POCUS)
- **20th century:** POCUS finds its way into medicine, academia, and into the hands of several properly trained practitioners, not limited to any single body system or chief complaint.
  - Ultrasound is now a vital component of bedside care throughout the United States.
  - POCUS is largely becoming the standard of care adhering to evidence based practice guidelines and recommendations that meets reimbursement criteria as set forth by insurers and the Centers for Medicare and Medicaid.

## CLINICAL APPLICATIONS

POCUS is useful in a multitude of patient presentations and can aid management decisions. POCUS can help identify the following:

- **Head, eyes, ears, nose, and throat (HEENT)**
  - Cranial
    - Intracranial pressure monitoring
    - Midline shift
  - Ocular
    - Lens dislocation
    - Retinal detachment
    - Vitreous hemorrhage
    - Optic nerve sheath diameter
    - Foreign body

- Neck
  - Thyroid
  - Lymph nodes
- **Cardiovascular**
  - Left ventricular function
  - Left ventricular hypertrophy
  - Wall motion abnormalities
  - Pericardial fluid
  - Cardiac standstill
  - Abdominal aortic aneurysm
  - Deep vein thrombosis
- **Respiratory**
  - Pneumothorax
  - Pulmonary effusion
  - Pneumonia or consolidation
- **Gastrointestinal (GI)**
  - Hydronephrosis
  - Cholelithiasis
  - Appendicitis
  - Intussusception
- **Genitourinary (GU)**
  - Testicular torsion
  - Renal calculi
  - Hydronephrosis
- **Obstetrical**
  - Measurement of gestational age
  - Fetal heart tones
  - Ectopic pregnancy
  - Intrauterine pregnancy
  - Bleeding in the first trimester
- **Endocrine**
  - Thyroid nodules
- **Musculoskeletal (MSK)**
  - Joint effusions
  - Dislocations
  - Fractures
  - Tendon abnormalities
  - Osteoarthritis

- **Skin**
  - Soft tissue infection
  - Cellulitis
  - Abscess
  - Foreign body
  - Fournier gangrene

## PROCEDURAL USE OF POINT-OF-CARE ULTRASOUND

- **HEENT**
  - Peritonsillar abscess
- **Airway**
  - Endotracheal tube (ETT) tube placement confirmation
  - Surgical airway
- **Cardiac**
  - Thoracentesis
  - Pericardiocentesis
- **Vascular access**
  - Central venous access
  - Peripheral vein access
  - Arterial cannulation
- **GI**
  - Paracentesis
- **GU**
  - Bladder aspiration
- **MSK**
  - Arthrocentesis
  - Reductions
  - Hematoma block
  - Foreign body removal
- **Neurological**
  - Lumbar puncture
- **Soft tissue**
  - Incision and drainage

## PROVIDER TRAINING

- Initial training largely occurs in the academic setting, fellowship, residency, continuing medical education, or workshops followed by a period of supervision
- Additional aids in training
  - Simulation
  - Internet-based

- Virtual reality
- Mobile device applications

## WHAT DOES THE EVIDENCE SAY?

- Cost-effective and safe
- Nonionizing radiation
- Portable
- Expedited decision making
- Improved patient satisfaction
- Improved procedural outcomes
  - Internal jugular venous cannulation first attempt success may improve by 57%.
  - Randomized trials show ultrasound guidance versus landmark guidance for paracentesis demonstrate success rates from 65% to 95%.
- Decreased postprocedural complications
  - POCUS for internal jugular venous cannulation reduced the rate of overall complications by 71%.
  - Systematic reviews show a significantly lower risk of pneumothorax following ultrasound-guided thoracentesis.

## WHAT IS THE FUTURE OF ULTRASOUND?

With the emergence of artificial intelligence in healthcare, POCUS makes auscultation, palpation, and a standard physical exam seem archaic. Moving beyond the boundaries of the stethoscope for real-time physiological evaluation introduces a new paradigm in our approach to patient care that is largely adopted as the standard of care (Osterwalkder et al., 2023). POCUS will continue to advance outside the healthcare setting and into our patients' hands, improve the safety of invasive surgical procedures, and  provide real-time diagnostic data in an expeditious manner reducing delays in patient care. (National Institute of Biomedical Imaging and Bioengineering, 2023).

- **POCUS providers diagnose and treat patients in real time**
  - Emergency medicine
  - Critical care
  - Outpatient
  - Urgent care
  - Emergency medical services (EMS)
  - Flight teams
- **POCUS expansion**
  - Internal medicine
  - Anesthesiology
  - Primary care
  - Specialties

- Cardiology/Pulmonology
- Dermatology
- GI
- Orthopedics
  - Ambulatory surgery centers
  - Patient homes
  - Digital apps
- **Utilization**
  - Providers
    - To aid in answering clinical questions and procedures
  - Nurses
    - Peripheral intravenous (PIV) catheter placement
  - EMS
    - PIV placement
    - ETT placement confirmation
    - Cardiac standstill
- **US devices will become more advanced, portable, accessible, and intuitive**
- **POCUS summary of clinical application**

  - Expedites plan of care
  - Improves workflow
  - Decreases procedural complications
  - Improves reimbursement meeting benchmark criteria
  - Standard of care

## BIBLIOGRAPHY

National Institute of Biomedical Imaging and Bioengineering. (2023). *Ultrasound*. Retrieved December 5, 2024, from https://www.nibib.nih.gov/science-education/science-topics/ultrasound
Osterwalkder, J., Polyzogopoulou, E., & Hoffmann, B. (2023). Point-of-care-ultrasound history, current and evolving clinical concepts in emergency medicine. *Medicine (Kaunas), 59*(12), 2179. https://doi.org/10.3390/medicina59122179

# CHAPTER 2

# ULTRASOUND PHYSICS AND FUNDAMENTALS

Marlen Alvarez and Kelli Craven

## FREQUENCY, WAVELENGTH, RESOLUTION, ATTENUATION

- **Frequency:** number of complete cycles per second, measured in hertz
- **Wavelength:** distance traveled during one cycle
  - Expressed in units of distance (m, cm, mm, etc.)
- **Resolution:** ability to discriminate between objects close together in space (spatial) or time (temporal)
  - Spatial Resolution
    - **Axial:** measures distance along a line that is parallel to the ultrasound beam
      - Usually unaffected by depth of imaging
      - Diminished dependency on beam width
    - **Lateral:** measures distance between objects lying side by side, or perpendicular to the beam
      - Heavily affected by depth of imaging and width of ultrasound beam
  - **Temporal Resolution:** ability to visualize moving objects
    - Measured in hertz
    - Used to scan multiple successive frames
    - Observes movement of an object throughout time
- **Attenuation:** loss of intensity and amplitude as sound waves travel through a medium

## PIEZOELECTRIC ENERGY AND HERTZ

- **Piezoelectric energy:** energy created by piezoelectric crystals
  - Crystals produce sound waves and when the sound waves return, they cause the crystals to vibrate, creating energy
- **Hertz**
  - Unit of measurement for frequency
  - One hertz represents one cycle per second which equates to one per second in radiology.

See Figure 2.1

> The anatomy of the ultrasound probe seen in Figure 2.1 is what allows the transducer to echo sound waves and reflect them back to the transducer through piezoelectric crystals. Using the speed of sound, the echoes returning to the transducer are measured at intervals along the path of the beam producing a 2-D image on the ultrasound screen (National Institute of Biomedical Imaging and Bioengineering, 2023).

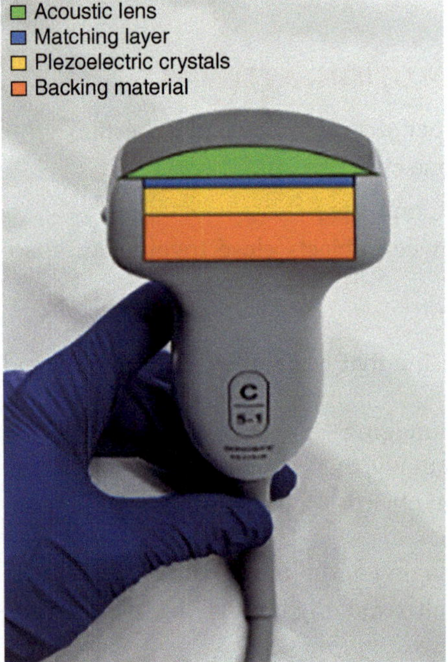


**Figure 2.1.** Anatomy of the ultrasound probe.

*Source:* Photo courtesy of Marlen Alvarez, DNP, FNP-C, ENP-C. Used with permission.

## IMAGE GENERATION

- **Gain**
  - Uniform amplification of the ultrasonic signal of returning echo
  - Functions as an amplifier
  - Makes image brighter or darker
- **Near field/far field**
  - **Near field:** cylindrical area of beam after leaving transducer
    - Length depends on width of transducer
    - The wider the transducer the longer the near field
    - Top half of the image

- **Far field:** when the beam begins to diverge
  - ○ Bottom half of the image

See Figure 2.2

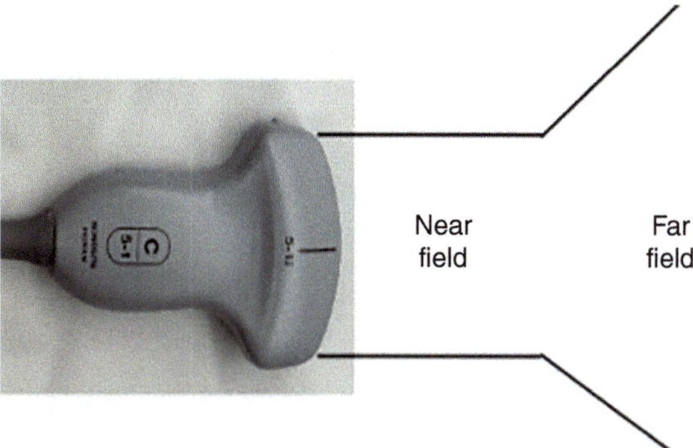


**Figure 2.2.** Ultrasound beam profile.
*Source:* Photo courtesy of Marlen Alvarez, DNP, FNP-C, ENP-C. Used with permission.

## IMAGING PLANES

- **Sagittal/longitudinal**
  - Scanning in a plane parallel to the structure
  - Probe marker pointing cephalad

See Figure 2.3

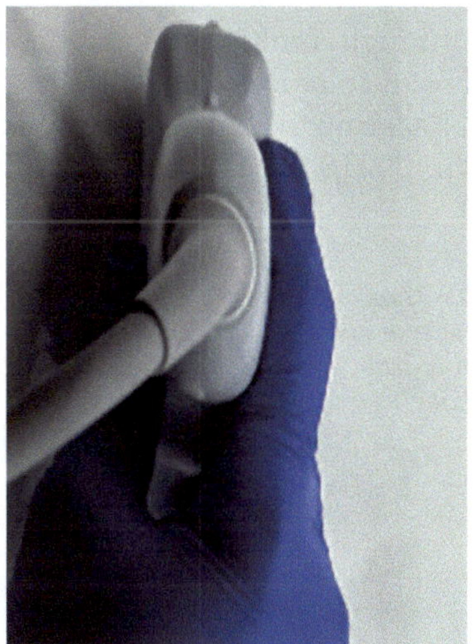

**Figure 2.3.** Longitudinal position (marker dot toward patient's head).
*Source:* Photo courtesy of Marlen Alvarez, DNP, FNP-C, ENP-C. Used with permission.

- ■ **Transverse**
  - • Scanning in a plane perpendicular to the structure
  - • Probe marker pointing to patient's right

See Figure 2.4

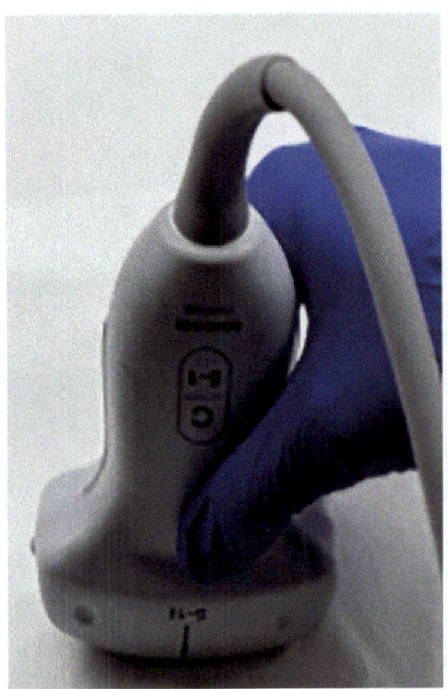

**Figure 2.4.** Transverse position (marker dot toward scanner's left).
*Source:* Photo courtesy of Marlen Alvarez, DNP, FNP-C, ENP-C. Used with permission.

## SUMMARY

Ultrasound technology continues to advance through multiple modalities. Application of new technology using new functions of color doppler, elastography, and smart glasses that overlay the ultrasound image on the field of view will revolutionize use of ultrasound (Osterwalkder et al., 2023).

## BIBLIOGRAPHY

National Institute of Biomedical Imaging and Bioengineering. (2023). *Ultrasound.* Retrieved December 5, 2024, from https://www.nibib.nih.gov/science-education/science-topics/ultrasound

Osterwalkder, J., Polyzogopoulou, E., & Hoffmann, B. (2023). Point-of-care-ultrasound history, current and evolving clinical concepts in emergency medicine. *Medicine (Kaunas), 59*(12), 2179. https://doi.org/10.3390/medicina59122179

# CHAPTER 3

# BASICS OF TRANSDUCERS, SCANNING MODES, AND ARTIFACT

Marlen Alvarez and Kelli Craven

## TRANSDUCER CHARACTERISTICS

- **Linear**
  - High frequency (5–15 MHz), high resolution
  - Linear footprint
  - Rectangular screen profile
  - Superficial structures (e.g., vascular, musculoskeletal, nerve, soft tissue imaging)
  - Max depth 9 cm
- **Phased Array**
  - Low frequency (1–5 MHz), medium range resolution
  - Triangular footprint
  - Pie-shaped screen profile
  - Optimal for cardiac, lung, and transcranial imaging
  - Max depth 35 cm
- **Curvilinear**
  - Low frequency (2–5 MHz)
  - Convex footprint
  - C-shaped screen profile
  - Deep penetration, low resolution
  - Used for deep structures such as abdominal, Focused Assessment with Sonography in Trauma (FAST) exams, and obstetric imaging
  - Max depth 30 cm
- **Endocavitary**
  - High frequency (8–13 MHz), high resolution
  - Microconvex footprint
  - C-shaped screen profile
  - Primarily used for transvaginal and transrectal imaging
  - Max depth 13 cm

See Figure 3.1

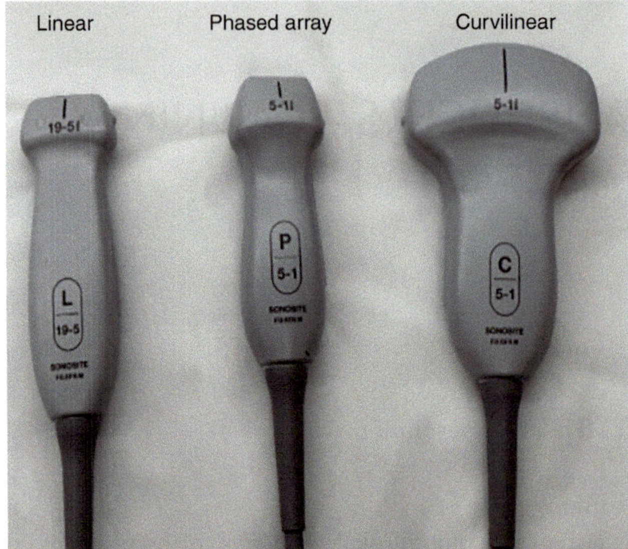


**Figure 3.1.** Types of transducers (not shown intracavitary).
*Source:* Photo courtesy of Marlen Alvarez, DNP, FNP-C, ENP-C. Used with permission.

## SCANNING MODES

- **B-Mode or 2D mode**
  - The standard scanning mode to begin each scan
  - Two-dimensional ultrasound image
  - Graphs the amplitude of reflected US waves on a grayscale
- **M-Mode or "Motion" mode**
  - One dimensional analysis
  - Movement over time and distance
  - Must use the M-mode cursor line over target structures
  - Useful for
    - Cardiac valves and wall motion
    - Fetal heart tones
    - Lung sliding in pneumothorax detection ("seashore sign" versus "barcode sign")
    - Vascular collapsibility
- **Doppler Settings**
  - Spectral Doppler
    - Velocity of blood flow over time as a waveform graph
    - Continuous
      - Used for high-velocity flow assessment, e.g., aortic stenosis and evaluating valvular regurgitation

- ○ Pulse wave
  - – Precise measurement of flow velocity at a specific location
  - – Blood velocity through left ventricular outflow tract
- Color Doppler
  - ○ Displays direction and velocity of flow
  - ○ Red depicts movement toward the transducer
    - – **R**ed = **R**eturn
  - ○ Blue depicts movement away from the transducer
    - – **B**lue = **B**ye
- Power Doppler = Low flow states
  - ○ Heart valve defects
  - ○ Congenital heart disease
  - ○ Arterial occlusion
  - ○ Stenosis of an artery
  - ○ Deep vein thrombosis
  - ○ Venous insufficiency
  - ○ Must use the color Doppler box
    - – Focus on area of interest
  - ○ Adjust the velocity rate
    - – High, medium or low

## TYPES OF ARTIFACT

■ **Reverberation**
- Occurs when the US beam encounters two highly reflective layers
- Screen appearance
  - ○ Bright hyperechoic lines parallel to one another
- Example
  - ○ A-lines in normal pleural assessment
- Tip to avoid reverberation
  - ○ Change transducer angle
    - – Tilting
  - ○ Decrease gain

■ **Shadowing**
- Occurs when dense structures completely absorb or reflect sound waves, creating a dark shadow underneath the hyperechoic appearing structure
- Seen with highly dense structures
  - ○ Bones
  - ○ Gallstones
- Tip to avoid shadowing
  - ○ Change transducer angle

■ **Mirroring**
- Highly reflective surface between the transducer and area of interest
- Duplicate image created on the opposite side
- Most commonly seen in pleural or liver imaging, where the diaphragm acts as a reflective surface, creating a false "mirror" of the liver above it
- Tip to avoid mirroring
  - Change scanning angle
  - Change scanning plane

■ **Edge**
- Refractive artifact
- Occurs at lateral edges of a curved boundary
  - Commonly occurs at the edges of cystic structures (e.g., bladder, gallbladder)
- Appears as thin hypoechoic line
- Tip to avoid edge
  - Change transducer angle

## BIBLIOGRAPHY

123 Sonography, (n.d.). *1.6.3 image resolution.* https://123sonography.com/ebook/image-resolution

American College of Emergency Physicians. (2020). *Sonoguide,* https://www.acep.org/sonoguide/basic/ultrasound-physics-and-technical-facts-for-the-beginner

Baad, M., Lu, F., Reiser, R., & Paushter, D. (2017). Clinical significance of US artifacts. *RadioGraphics, 37*(5), 1408–1423. https://doi.org/10.1148/rg.2017160175

Bell, D. (2021a). *Piezoelectric effect.* Radiopaedia, https://radiopaedia.org/articles/piezoelectric-effect

Bell, D. (2021b). *Hertz.* Radiopaedia, https://radiopaedia.org/articles/hertz

Bornemann, P., & Barreto, T. (2018, August 15). Point-of-care ultrasonography in family medicine. *American Family Physician, 98*(4), 200–202. https://www.aafp.org/pubs/afp/issues/2018/0815/p200.html

Brass, P., Hellmich, M., Kolodziej, L., Schick, G., & Smith, A. F. (2015, January 9). Ultrasound guidance versus anatomical landmarks for internal jugular vein catheterization. *Cochrane Database of Systematic Reviews, 1*(1), CD006962. https://doi.org/10.1002/14651858

Campos, Arlene. (June 28, 2024). *Grey scale imaging (ultrasound). Radiopaedia.* https://radiopaedia.org/articles/grey-scale-imaging-ultrasound?lang=us

Choi, W., Cho, Y. S., Ha, Y. R., Oh, J. H., Lee, H., Kang, B. S., Kim, Y. W., Koh, C. Y., Lee, J. H., Jung, E., Sohn, Y., Kim, H. B., Kim, S. J., Kim, H., Suh, D., Lee, D. H., Hong, J. Y., Lee, W. W., & Society Emergency and Critical Care Imaging. (2023, December). Role of point-of-care ultrasound in critical care and emergency medicine: Update and future perspective. *Clinical and Experimental Emergency Medicine, 10*(4), 363–381. https://doi.org/10.15441/ceem.23.101

Critical Care North Hampton. *Physics of ultrasound.* https://criticalcarenorthampton.com/physics-of-ultrasound/

FUSIC-SY. *Ultrasound physics.* https://fusic-sy.co.uk/education/ultrasound-physics

Galdamez, A. L. (2019). *The evolving role of ultrasound in emergency medicine.* IntechOpen. https://doi.org/10.5772/intechopen.74777

Gill, B. (2019). *Ultrasound probes: The break down.* Probo Medical. https://www.probomedical.com/learn/blog/ultrasound-probes-the-break-down/

Gordon, C. E., Feller-Kopman, D., Balk, E. M., & Smetana, G. W. (2010). Pneumothorax following thoracentesis: A systematic review and meta-analysis. *Archives of Internal Medicine, 170*(4), 332–339. https://doi.org/10.1001/archinternmed.2009.548

Hashim, A., Tahir, M. J., Ullah, I., Asghar, M. S., Siddiqi, H., & Yousaf, Z. (2021, November 2). The utility of point of care ultrasonography (POCUS). *Annals of Medicine and Surgery (London), 71*, 102982. https://doi.org/10.1016/j.amsu.2021.102982

MXR: The Imaging Solutions Company. https://mxrimaging.com/Axial-Lateral-and-Temporal-Resolution-in-Ultrasoun

Nazeer, S. R., Dewbre, H., & Miller, A. H. (2005). Ultrasound-assisted paracentesis performed by emergency physicians vs the traditional technique: A prospective, randomized study *The American Journal of Emergency Medicine, 23*(3), 363–367. https://doi.org/10.1016/j.ajem.2004.11.001

POCUS 101. *Ultrasound machine basics-knobology, probes, and modes*. https://www.pocus101.com/ultrasound-machine-basics-knobology-probes-and-modes/#Linear_Ultrasound_Probe

Radiology Café. *Producing an ultrasound beam* https://www.radiologycafe.com/frcr-physics-notes/ultrasound-imaging/producing-an-ultrasound-beam/

Rice, J. A., Brewer, J., Speaks, T., Choi, C., Lahsaei, P., & Romito, B. T. (2021, December 15). The POCUS consult: How point of care ultrasound helps guide medical decision making. *International Journal of General Medicine, 14*, 9789–9806. https://doi.org/10.2147/IJGM

Saul, T., Siadecki, S. D., Berkowitz, R., Rose, G., Matilsky, D., & Sauler, A. (2015). M-mode ultrasound applications for the emergency medicine physician. *The Journal of Emergency Medicine, 49*(5), 686–692. https://doi.org/10.1016/j.jemermed.2015.06.059

Soni, N. J., Arntfield, R., & Kory, P. (2020). *Point of care ultrasound* (2nd ed.). Elsevier

Walls, R. M., Hockberger, R. S., Gausche-Hill, M., Erickson, T. B., & Wilcox, S. R. (2023). *Rosen's emergency medicine: Concepts and clinical practice*. Elsevier.

Wierman, D. (2019). Understanding gain in ultrasound. *E.I. Medical Imaging*. https://www.eimedical.com/blog/understanding-gain-in-ultrasound

Zander, D., Hüske, S., Hoffmann, B., Cui, X. W., Dong, Y., Lim, A., Jenssen, C., Löwe, A., Koch, J. B. H., & Dietrich, C. F. (2020, June). Ultrasound image optimization ("Knobology"): B-mode. *Ultrasound International Open, 6*(1), E14–E24. https://doi.org/10.1055/a-1223-1134

# CHAPTER 4

# EXTENDED FOCUS ASSESSMENT WITH SONOGRAPHY IN TRAUMA (E-FAST EXAM)

Adriana De La Rue

## INTRODUCTION

- **E-FAST**: extended focused assessment with sonography in trauma
  - Includes pleural assessment for pneumothorax
- Standard of care in diagnostic evaluation of the trauma patient or hemodynamically unstable patient of unclear etiology
- Advanced trauma life support (ATLS) guidelines, surgeons, emergency providers, American College of Emergency Physicians, and American Academy of Emergency Nurse Practitioners recommend and support use of point-of-care ultrasound E-FAST in the appropriate setting
- **Six views**: cardiac, right upper quadrant (RUQ), left upper quadrant (LUQ), pelvic/bladder, right thoracic intercostal and left thoracic intercostal
- More sensitive than plain chest radiography for identification of pneumothorax
- High specificity greater than 98% for detecting hemopericardium and hemoperitoneum, but its sensitivity (85%–95%) varies depending on fluid volume and operator experience (Rowland-Fisher & Reardon, 2021).

See Tables 4.1 and 4.2 for information on indications and differentials.

**Table 4.1** Indications

| Blunt or penetrating trauma | Chest pain |
| --- | --- |
| Dyspnea | Hemodynamic instability |
| Abdominal pain | Vaginal bleeding |
| Hematuria | Back pain |

**Table 4.2** Differentials

| Cardiac tamponade | Pneumothorax/hemothorax | Pleural effusion |
| --- | --- | --- |
| Pleural consolidation | AAA | Organ injury |
| Peritoneal free fluid | IUP | Ectopic pregnancy |

AAA, abdominal aortic aneurysm; IUP, intrauterine pregnancy.

# IMAGE ACQUISITION

See Figure 4.1

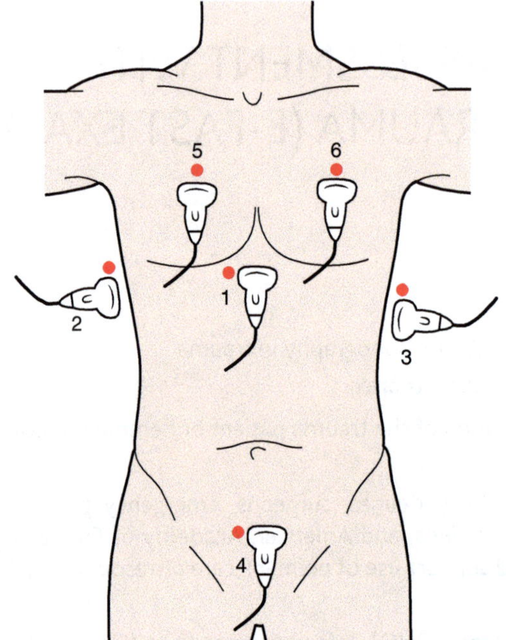

1) Subxiphoid cardiac (marker dot towards scanner's left)
2) RUQ (marker dot towards patient's head)
3) LUQ (marker dot towards patient's head)
4) Pelvic/bladder transverse (marker dot towards scanner's left)
   Longitudinal (marker dot towards patient's head)
5) Right 2nd intercostal space (marker dot towards patient's head)
6) Left 2nd intercostal space (marker dot towards patient's head)

**Figure 4.1.** E-FAST transducer positions.

- ■ **Transducer**
  - **Curvilinear:** entire exam
  - **Phased array:** entire exam
  - **Linear:** thoracic views ONLY
  - Best for pneumothorax detection due to higher resolution of pleural sliding
  - Select FAST/E-FAST preset on ultrasound machine

### PRO TIP

Utilize same probe throughout exam to improve speed and efficiency.

- ■ **Hand placement**
  - Hold the probe in your dominant hand with the ultrasound machine within reach of your non-dominant hand

- ○ **Cardiac:** hold like a computer mouse, index finger on top of transducer
  - ○ **RUQ/LUQ:** hold the probe in palm of your hand, cupping fingers around base.
  - ○ **Pelvic:** hold like a pencil or "okay" sign
  - ○ **Thoracic:** hold like a pencil.
- ■ **Technique**
  - Transverse view
    - ○ Probe indicator always to the patient's right
  - Longitudinal view
    - ○ Probe indicator pointing cephalad
  - Cardiac
    - ○ Place probe directly below xiphoid process and hold firm direct pressure inward and upward until heart is brought into view.
    - ○ Evaluate for fluid within the pericardial sac.

**PRO TIP**

Must differentiate between anechoic fluid and fat pad.

- ○ Cardiac tamponade: obtain additional cardiac views and inferior vena cava (IVC)
- RUQ
  - ○ Place probe between ribs 8 and 11 in midaxillary line
  - ○ Evaluate inferior kidney, caudal tip of liver, Morison's pouch (hepato-renal recess), suprahepatic (diaphragm) while fanning the probe from anterior to posterior

**PRO TIP**

Lack of mirroring of the liver is concerning for pleural effusion or hemothorax.

- LUQ
  - ○ Place probe between ribs 8 and 11.
  - ○ Evaluate splenorenal recess, while fanning the probe from anterior to posterior.

**PRO TIPS**

Knuckles to the bed, pointing toward the head.

Spine sign (spine visualized above diaphragm) is concerning for pleural effusion or hemothorax.

- Pelvic
  - ○ Place probe halfway between umbilicus and pubic symphysis
  - ○ Longitudinal view: probe marker to patient's head, locate bladder while fanning the probe from right to left
    - – Evaluate fluid superior and posterior to bladder

- Transverse view: probe marker to the patient's right, locate bladder and fan the probe superiorly and inferiorly

**PRO TIP**

If unable to locate bladder, identify pubic shadow.

- Thoracic Views
- Second intercostal space, midclavicular line bilaterally
- Longitudinal view: locate hyperechoic line (pleural line)
  - Evaluate for lung sliding between parietal and visceral pleural, often described as "ants on a log" or "shimmering'
  - Evaluate for lung "point": an area of pleural sliding meets an area stationary presentation and no evidence of lung sliding

**PRO TIP**

Confirm lung sliding in M-Mode.
- Normal Lung Sliding.
  - "Seashore" sign or "sky meets beach" = sandy beach [lung slide] below pleural line meets barcode [no lung slide] above pleural line.
- Absent Lung Sliding.
  - Barcode = bad (concerning for pneumothorax), barcode above and below pleural line.

## ANATOMY/IMAGES

■ **Cardiac**

See Figure 4.2

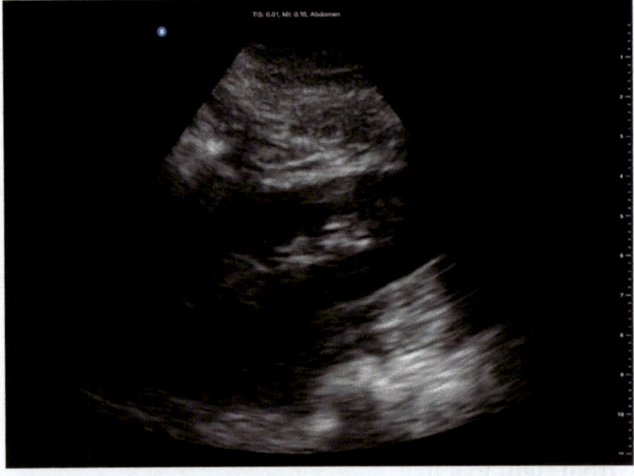

**Figure 4.2.** Normal hepatorenal space.

*Source:* Used with permission. Image courtesy of Dr. Kelli Craven.

## ▪ RUQ View

See Figure 4.3

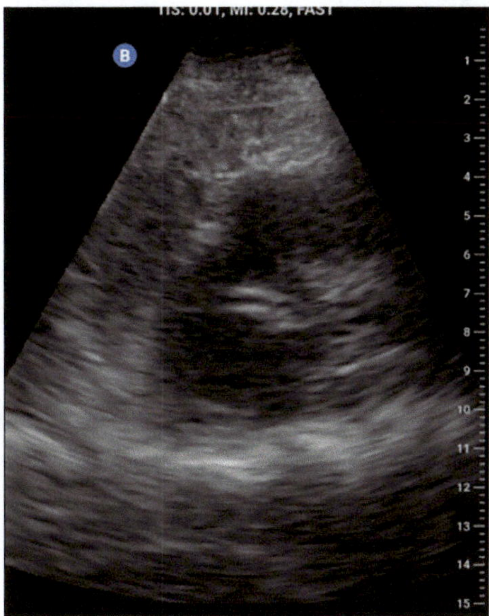

**Figure 4.3.** Normal splenorenal space.
*Source:* Used with permission. Image courtesy of Dr. Kelli Craven.

## ▪ LUQ (Splenorenal)

See Figure 4.4

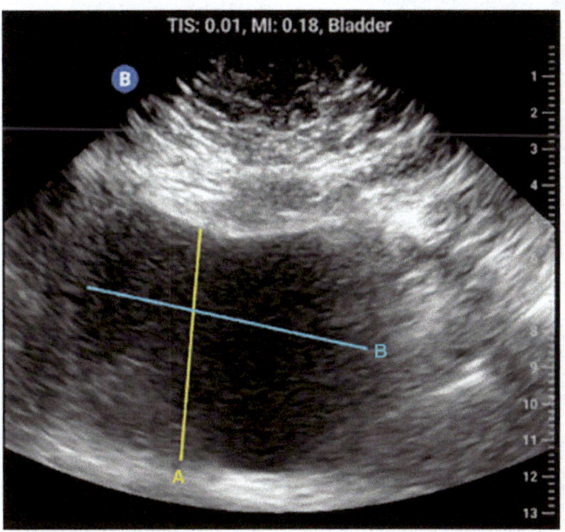

**Figure 4.4.** Normal bladder transverse.
*Source:* Used with permission. Image courtesy of Dr. Kelli Craven.

## ▪ Pelvic

See Figure 4.5

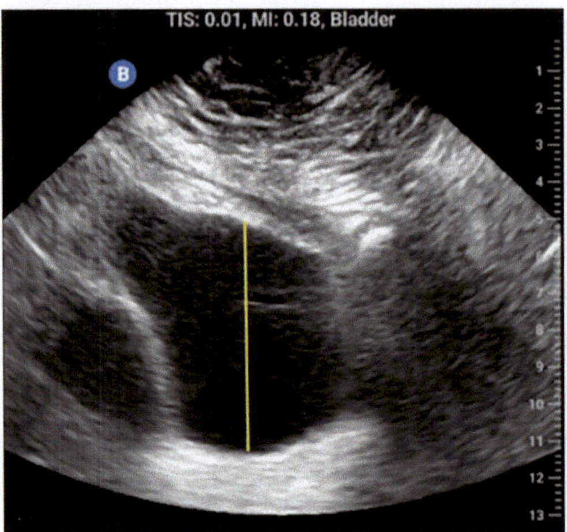

**Figure 4.5.** Normal bladder longitudinal.

*Source:* Used with permission. Image courtesy of Dr. Kelli Craven.

## ▪ Thoracic

See Figure 4.6

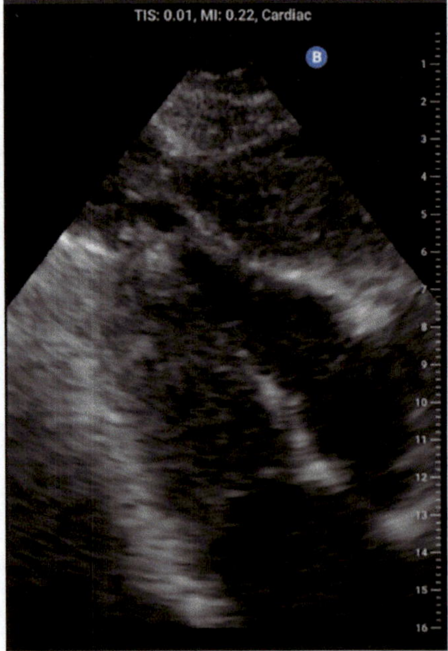

**Figure 4.6.** Subxiphoid pericardial window.

*Source:* Used with permission. Image courtesy of Dr. Kelli Craven.

## ■ Other

Figures 4.7 through 4.9 depict pericardial effusion with pulmonary effusion noted in the parasternal short axis, abnormal lung findings with moderate pleural effusion, and a normal IVC view.

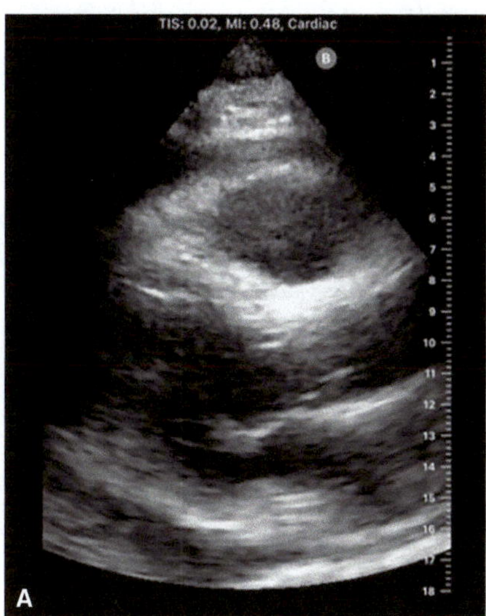
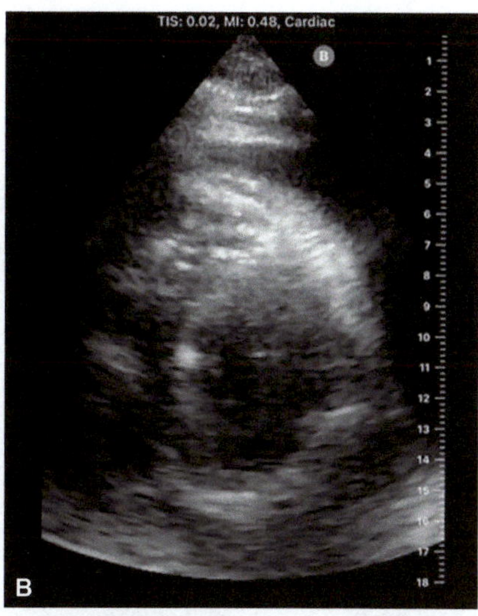

**Figure 4.7. (A)** Parasternal long axis in cardiac preset that demonstrates a moderate to large pericardial effusion. **(B)** Parasternal short axis in cardiac preset that demonstrates a moderate to large pericardial effusion.

*Source:* Sundberg, J. E., & Mehta A. (2022). A brisk and life-saving diagnosis of pericardial effusion as the cause for recurrent dyspnea. *POCUS Journal, 7*(1), 124–126. https://doi.org/10.24908/pocus.v7i1.15162

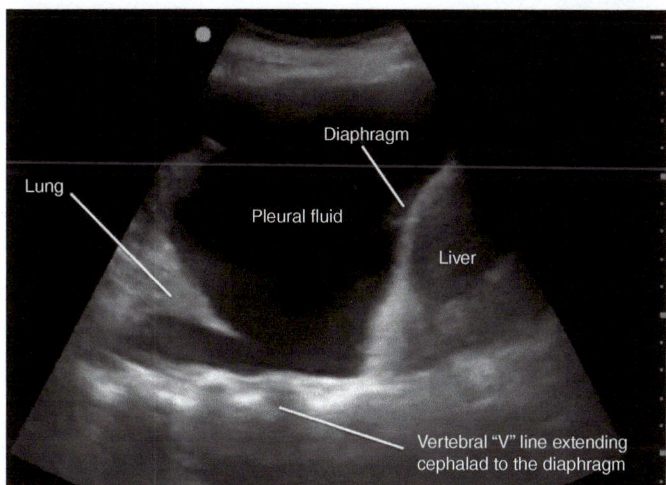


**Figure 4.8.** Abnormal lung finding with moderate pleural effusion noted.

*Source:* Atkinson, P., Milne, J., Loubani, O., & Verheul, G. (2012). The V-line: a sonographic aid for the confirmation of pleural fluid. *Critical Ultrasound Journal, 4,* 19. https://doi.org/10.1186/2036-7902-4-19

## INTERPRETATION

- Any sign of intraperitoneal free fluid constitutes a positive exam.
- Lung point (transition from sliding to absent sliding) is pathognomonic for pneumothorax
- The Barcode sign (M-mode) confirms absence of lung sliding.

See Figures 4.10 and 4.11 for images depicting "barcode" and "seashore" signs in lung sliding images.

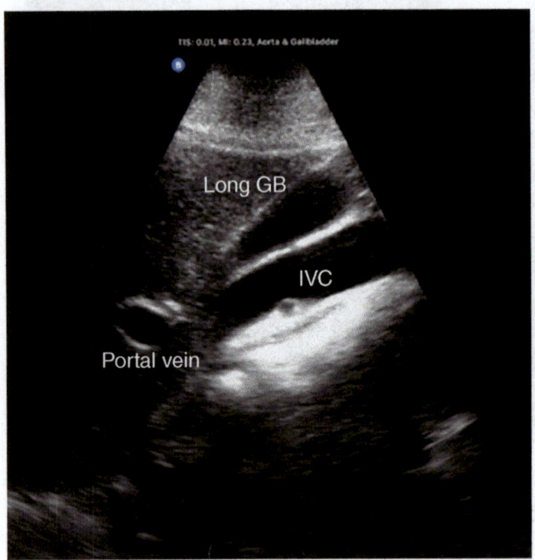


**Figure 4.9.** Normal inferior vena cava view.

*Source:* Used with permission. Image courtesy of Dr. Kelli Craven.

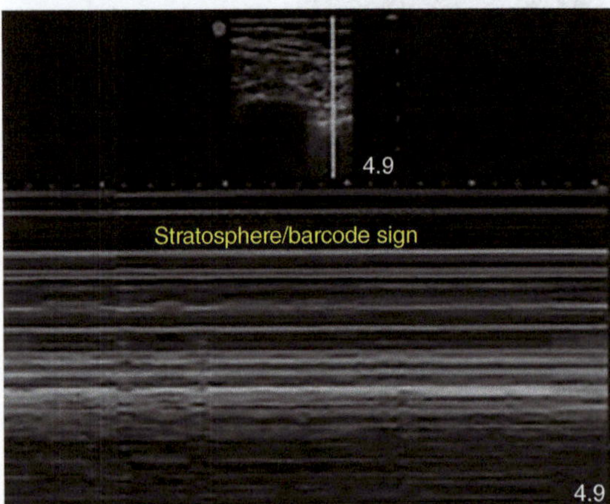


**Figure 4.10.** Absent lung sliding demonstrates "barcode" sign.

*Source:* Arora, D., Vadera, H., & Rath, A. (2024). E-FAST and abdominal ultrasound. In Bouarroudj, N., Cano, P. C., Fathil, S. B. M., & Hemamid, H. (Eds.) POCUS in critical care, anesthesia and emergency medicine. Springer. https://doi.org/10.1007/978-3-031-43721-2_12

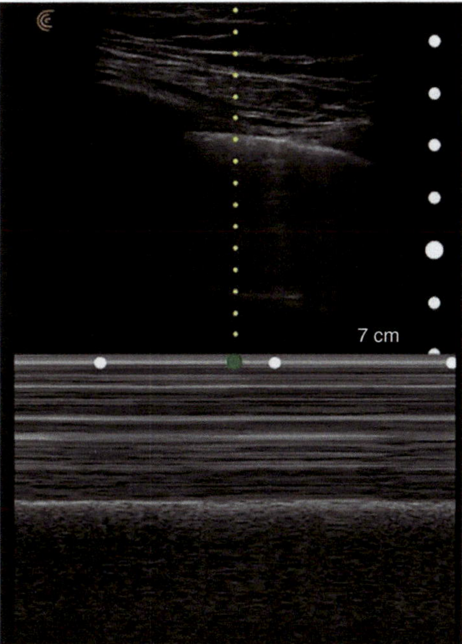

**Figure 4.11.** Normal lung sliding "seashore" sign.
*Source:* Clarius Mobile Health.

See Table 4.3

## Table 4.3 Summary of Pathologic Findings

| Condition | Ultrasound Findings |
| --- | --- |
| Pericardial effusion | Anechoic fluid within pericardial sac |
| Cardiac tamponade | Anechoic fluid within pericardial sac + right ventricular collapse + non-collapsible IVC |
| Free fluid in the abdomen | Anechoic fluid |
| Ascites | Large anechoic collections through abdomen |
| Ruptured ectopic pregnancy | Large anechoic collections through abdomen |
| Ruptured bladder | Large anechoic collections through abdomen and disruption of bladder wall |
| Urinary retention | Enlarged bladder with greater than 500 mL urine |
| Pneumothorax | Barcode sign<br>No lung sliding |
| Hemothorax | No mirroring on RUQ/LUQ views<br>Spine sign in RUQ/LUQ views |
| Pleural effusion | No mirroring in RUQ/LUQ views<br>Spine sign in RUQ/LUQ views |
| Fluid overload | B-lines on thoracic views |

IVC, inferior vena cava; LUQ, left upper quadrant; RUQ, right upper quadrant.

## PEARLS AND PITFALLS

- Troubleshooting cardiac view: Have the patient take a deep breath and hold for 5–10 seconds to bring the heart caudal.
- If the subxiphoid view is poor, consider a parasternal long axis view for pericardial fluid assessment.
- If gas (free air) is present in the abdomen and hindering views, hold pressure for about 1 minute.
- Repetition is key; complete exam in the same order every time
- Does not rule out retroperitoneal hemorrhage due to limited visibility, a negative scan does not rule out injury in pelvic or great vessel trauma.
- A minimum of 150 to 200 mL of free fluid is typically needed for ultrasound detection in the peritoneum, though smaller amounts may be visible in the hepatorenal or splenorenal recesses.
- Does not identify the source of hemorrhage

## VIDEOS

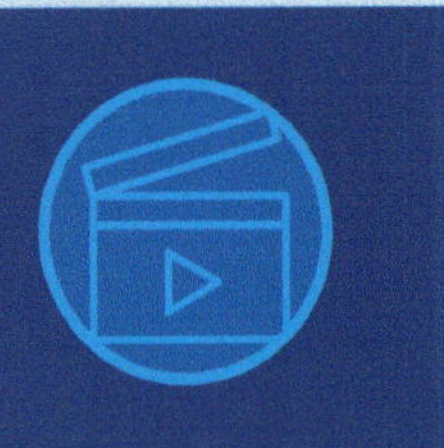

- Subxiphoid/Subcostal View
- Extended Focused Assessment With Sonography in Trauma (E-FAST) Exam
- Pleural Evaluation in Extended Focused Assessment With Sonography in Trauma (E-FAST) Exam

**To access the videos, please go to the List of Videos in the front matter.**

## BIBLIOGRAPHY


Avila, J. (2020, February). 5 min sono—EFAST. *Core Ultrasound.* https://coreultrasound.com/efast/

Habrat, D. (2003, December). How to do E-FAST examination. *Merck Manuals Professional Version.* https://www.merckmanuals.com/professional/critical-care-medicine/how-to-do-other-emergency-medicine-procedures/how-to-do-e-fast-examination

Pariyadath, M., & Snead, G. (n.d.). Emergency ultrasound in adults with abdominal and thoracic trauma. *UpToDate.* https://www.uptodate.com/contents/emergency-ultrasound-in-adults-with-abdominal-and-thoracic-trauma

Rowland-Fisher, A. & Reardon, R.F. (2021). E-FAST (Extended Focused Assessment with Sonography in Trauma). *American College of Emergency Physicians.* Retrieved August 28, 2024, from https://www.acep.org/sonoguide/basic/fast

Savoia, P., Jayanthi, S. K., & Chammas, M. C. (2023). Focused Assessment with Sonography for Trauma (FAST). *Journal of Medical Ultrasound, 31*(2), 101–106. https://doi.org/10.4103/jmu.jmu_12_23

White, S., Dihn, V., Ahn, J., Deschamps, J., Genobage, S., Lang, A., Lee, V., Tooma, D., & Krause, R. (n.d.). eFAST ultrasound exam made easy: Step by step guide. *Pocus101.* https://www.pocus101.com/efast-ultrasound-exam-made-easy-step-by-step-guide

Young, N., Luckett-Gatopoulos, S., Mohammed, M., Jordan, M., Ye, T., & Donaldson, R. (n.d.). EFAST exam. *WikiEM.* https://wikem.org/wiki/EFAST_exam

# CHAPTER 5

# ABDOMINAL AORTIC ANEURYSM

John Barrett

## INTRODUCTION

- Abdominal aortic aneurysms often found incidentally in 8% of the population and, if ruptured, have mortality rates as high as 80% (Marcaccio & Schermerhorn, 2021).

- AAA undiagnosed or untreated carries excessive mortality rates reaching 80%.

- Risk factors include male sex, older age, family history of AAA, and history of smoking (Marcaccio & Schermerhorn, 2021).

- With a technically adequate study, ultrasound has a sensitivity of 98% and specificity of 99% in detecting abdominal aortic aneurysms (Shaban et al., 2025).

- Most abdominal aortic aneurysms are below the level of the renal arteries (Shaw, Loree, & Oropallo, 2025).

- 94% of abdominal aortic aneurysms are fusiform; 6% are saccular (Karthaus, Tong, & Vahl, 2020)

See Tables 5.1 and 5.2 for information on indications and differentials.

**Table 5.1** Indications

| Abdominal pain | Flank pain | Back pain | Hypotension/shock |
|---|---|---|---|
| Pulsatile abdominal mass | Chest pain | Dyspnea | Syncope |

**Table 5.2** Differentials

| AAA | Appendicitis | Bowel obstruction/ perforation | Cholelithiasis/ cholecystitis | Diverticulitis | Ectopic pregnancy |
|---|---|---|---|---|---|
| Mesenteric ischemia | Superior vena cava syndrome | Nephrolithiasis | GERD | MI/ACS | Ascites/free air |

AAA, abdominal aortic aneurysm; ACS, acute coronary syndrome; GERD, gastroesophageal reflux disease; MI, myocardial infarction

## IMAGE ACQUISITION

- **Probe**

Curvilinear (see Figure 5.1)

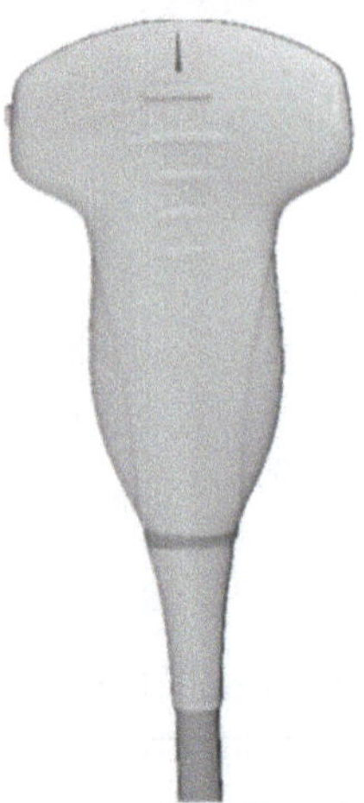

**Figure 5.1.** Curvilinear probe.

*Source:* Used with permission from John Barrett, DNP.

- **Hand placement**
  - Overhand grip with fingers wrapping around probe like a flashlight
- **Technique**
  - Transverse plane
    - Probe marker pointed to patient's right
    - Scan entirety of abdominal aorta from just below xyphoid process through iliac bifurcation near level of the umbilicus
  - Longitudinal plane
    - Probe marker pointed to patient's head
    - Scan entirety of abdominal aorta from just below xiphoid process through iliac bifurcation near level of the umbilicus
  - Measure at least 4 locations plus largest diameter
    - Transverse proximal aorta (@ celiac trunk)
    - Transverse mid aorta (@ superior mesenteric artery [SMA])
    - Transverse distal aorta (@ proximal to iliac bifurcation)
    - Longitudinal view of aorta
    - Measure outer wall to outer wall—do not mistake false lumen as entire aorta

## PRO TIPS

Use gentle, constant downward pressure to help move bowel aside.

If unable to view aorta, move probe slightly off midline and angle beam toward aorta.

## INTERPRETATION

- ≤3 cm = normal
- >3 cm = enlarged

See Figure 5.2 for normal aorta images and Figure 5.3 for abnormal aorta images.

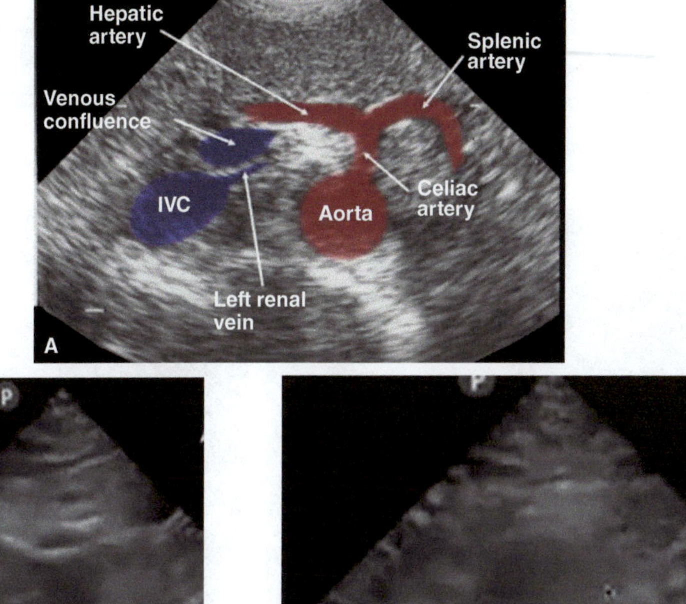


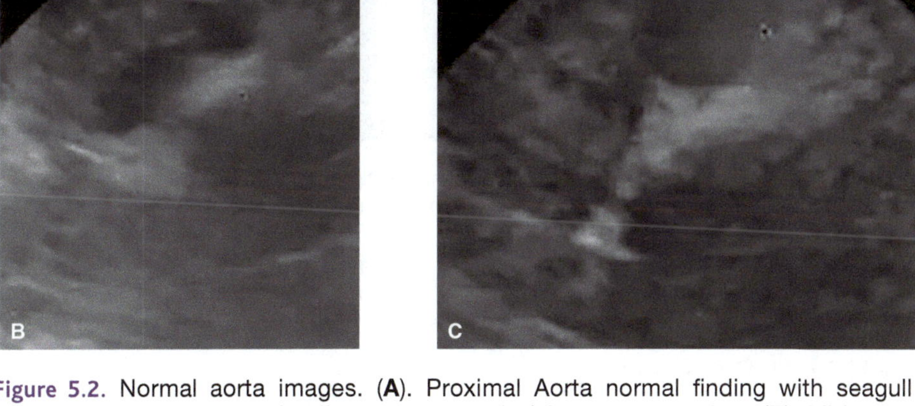


**Figure 5.2.** Normal aorta images. (**A**). Proximal Aorta normal finding with seagull sign (hepatic, splenic, and celiac artery complex) in transverse view. (**B**). Mid aorta in transverse view. Note the transverse colon just superior to the aorta and apply firm but gentle pressure to displace bowel gas. (**C**). Distal aorta in transverse view. (**D**). Longitudinal view of aorta. Note aorta is the large anechoic structure with superior mesenteric artery (SMA) just superior to the aorta.

*Source:* Dinh, V., & Tooma, D. (2019). Aorta ultrasound made easy. *POCUS 101 Tutorials.* Retrieved from https://www.pocus101.com/aorta-ultrasound-made-easy-step-by-step-guide/.

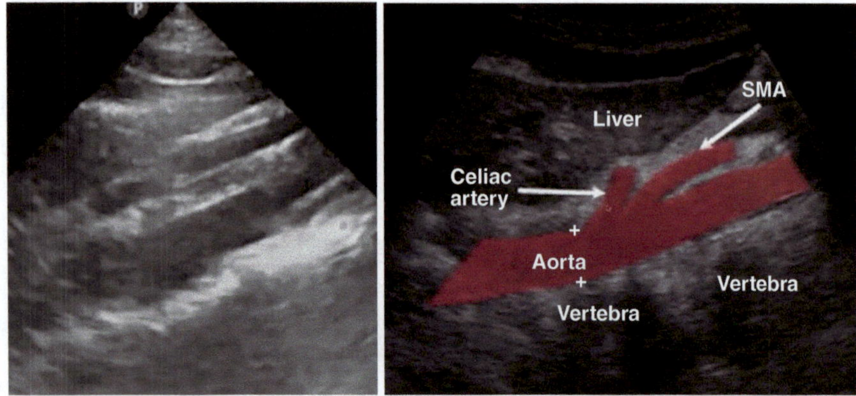



**Figure 5.2.** *(continued)*

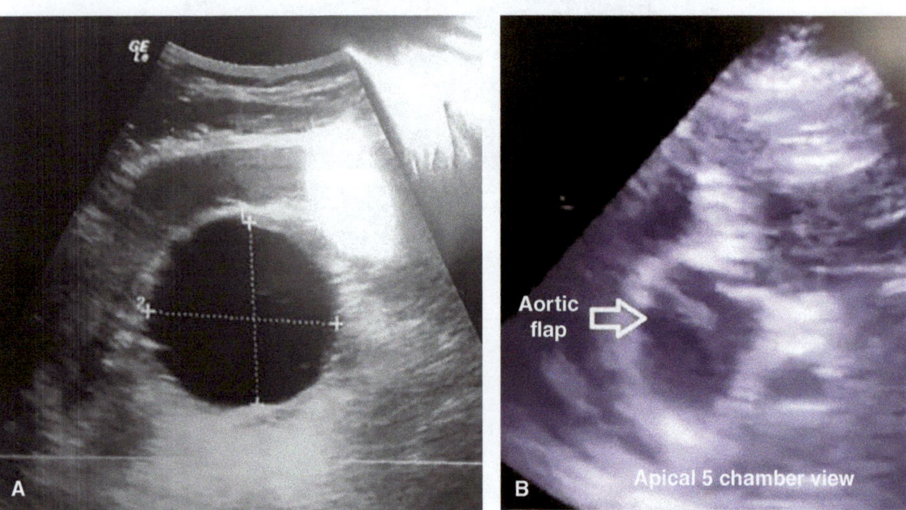



**Figure 5.3.** Abnormal aorta images. (**A**) Abdominal aortic aneurysm measuring 5.4 x 5.8 cm with peri-aortic hematoma. (**B**) Aortic intimal flap seen in apical five chamber view and parasternal short axis view.

*Source:* Khidir, M., Hanisah, N., Alwi, F., & Saim, A. (2019). Two cases of aortic emergency presenting with neurologic manifestations, aided by POCUS. *POCUS Journal*, 4(1), 9–12. https://pocusjournal.com/wp-content/uploads/2019/03/POCUSJ-2019_vol04_iss01p9-12.pdf

## PEARLS AND PITFALLS

- Bowel gas can obstruct view—gentle, constant downward pressure can help move bowel aside.
- Ensure measurement of the largest diameter outer wall to outer wall—one could mistake the inner wall of a thrombus for the aortic wall.
- Ultrasound is not sensitive enough to rule out aortic dissection.
- Do not mistake the inferior vena cava (IVC) for the aorta.
- Ensure visualization of branches of the aorta—e.g., celiac trunk, SMA.

## BIBLIOGRAPHY

American College of Emergency Physicians. (2021, October). *Emergency ultrasound imaging criteria compendium: Policy statement.* https://www.acep.org/siteassets/new-pdfs/policy-statements/emergency-ultrasound-imaging-criteria-compendium.pdf

Karthaus, E. G., Tong, T. M. L., & Vahl, A. (2020). Saccular abdominal aortic aneurysms: patient characteristics, clinical presentation, treatment, and outcomes in the Netherlands. *Journal of Vascular Surgery, 71*(2), 714. https://doi.org/10.1016/j.jvs.2019.11.008

Kuhn, M., Bonnin, R. L., Davey, M. J., Rowland, J. L., & Langlois, S. L. (2000). Emergency department ultrasound scanning for abdominal aortic aneurysm: accessible, accurate, and advantageous. *Annals of Emergency Medicine, 36*(3), 219–223. https://doi.org/10.1067/mem.2000.108616

Marcaccio, C. L., & Schermerhorn, M. L. (2021). Epidemiology of abdominal aortic aneurysms. *Seminars in Vascular Surgery, 34*(1), 29–37. https://doi.org/10.1053/j.semvascsurg.2021.02.004

Shaban, E. E., Yigit, Y., Alkahlout, B., Shaban, A., Shaban, A., Ponappan, B., Abdurabu, M., & Zaki, H. A. (2025). Enhancing clinical outcomes: Point of care ultrasound in the precision diagnosis and Management of Abdominal Aortic Aneurysms in emergency medicine: A systematic review and meta-analysis. *Journal of Clinical Ultrasound, 53*(2), 325–335. https://doi.org/10.1002/jcu.23850

Shaw, P. M., Loree, J., & Oropallo, A. (2025, January). Abdominal aortic aneurysm. In *StatPearls* [Internet]. StatPearls Publishing. https://www.ncbi.nlm.nih.gov/books/NBK470237/

# POINT-OF-CARE ULTRASOUND CARDIAC ECHOCARDIOGRAPHY

John Barrett

## INTRODUCTION

- Trained providers can rapidly estimate left ventricular (LV) ejection fraction (EF), right ventricular (RV) function, and intravascular volume status using point-of-care ultrasound (POCUS).
- Right ventricular dysfunction and dilation can be identified by POCUS.
- POCUS has a 90.4% to 98.9% sensitivity for detecting pericardial effusion.

See Tables 6.1 and 6.2 for indications and differentials.

**Table 6.1** Indications

| Chest Pain | Dyspnea/cough | Hypotension | Trauma |
|---|---|---|---|
| Hypoxemia | Cardiac arrest | Shock | Adventitious lung sounds |

**Table 6.2** Differentials

| Heart failure | ACS/MI | Pericardial effusion | Pleural effusion |
|---|---|---|---|
| Right heart strain | Pulmonary embolism | Pneumothorax | Pneumonia |

ACS, acute coronary syndrome; MI, myocardial infarction.

## IMAGE ACQUISITION

- **Probe**
  - Phased array
- **Hand placement**
  - Parasternal long axis (PLAX), parasternal short axis (PSSA), apical four-chamber (A4C)—hold probe like a pencil
  - Subxiphoid/subcostal view—overhand grip
- **Technique**

  - PLAX
    - Probe on anterior chest at the third to fifth intercostal space, just left of the sternum

- ○ Probe marker pointed toward left hip in FAST exam preset (cardiology preset = probe marker to right shoulder)
- ○ Left atrium, LV, RV, aorta, aortic and mitral valves should all be visible

See Figure 6.1 for an image depicting normal cardiac anatomy.

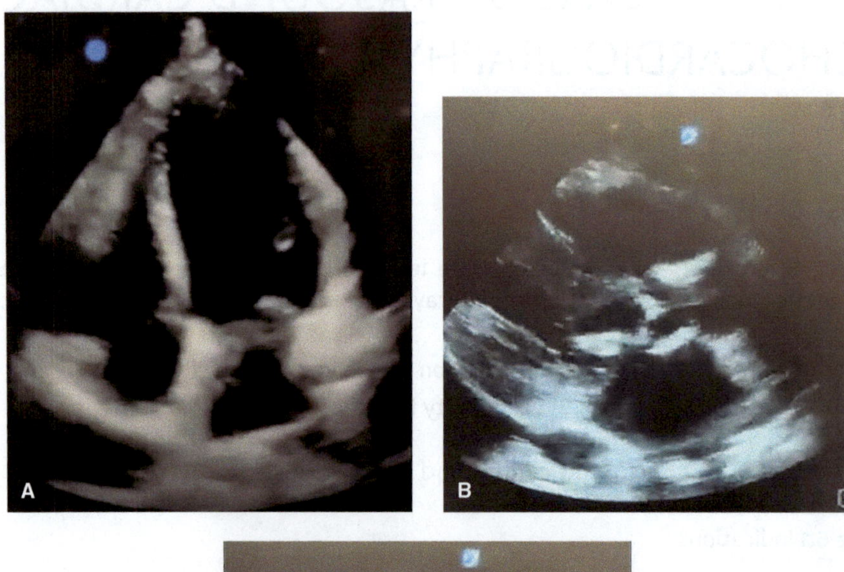

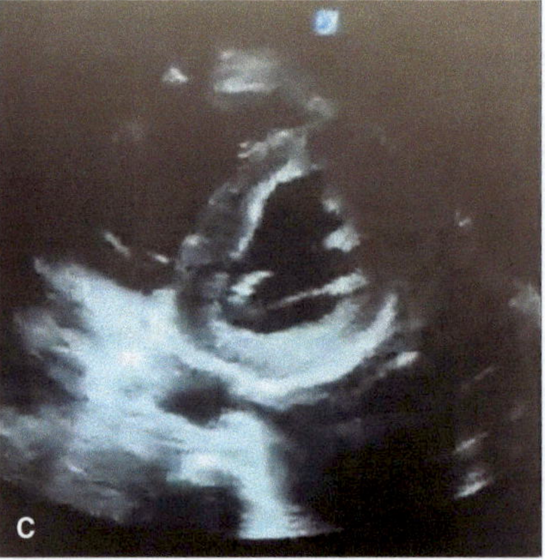

**Figure 6.1.** Normal cardiac anatomy (FAST preset not cardiac). (**A**) Normal cardiac apical 4 view in FAST preset. (**B**) Normal parasternal long axis view in cardiac present. (**C**) Normal cardiac parasternal short axis view in cardiac preset.

*Source:* Part A courtesy of Meg Petzy. Parts B and C courtesy of Ari Chaskes.

- PSSA
  - ○ From the PLAX window, rotate probe clockwise 90° with probe marker facing right hip (cardiac preset = left shoulder).
  - ○ Angle beam down through mitral valve to visualize "fish mouth" appearance of papillary muscles.

- A4C
  - Probe marker pointed to the right hip (cardiac preset = left shoulder)
  - Place probe at the point of maximal impulse, usually the fifth intercostal space, midclavicular line
  - Rotate patient into partial left lateral decubitus position for better visualization

**PRO TIP**

A moderator band is only seen in the RV.

See Figure 6.2 for images depicting normal anatomy moderator band.

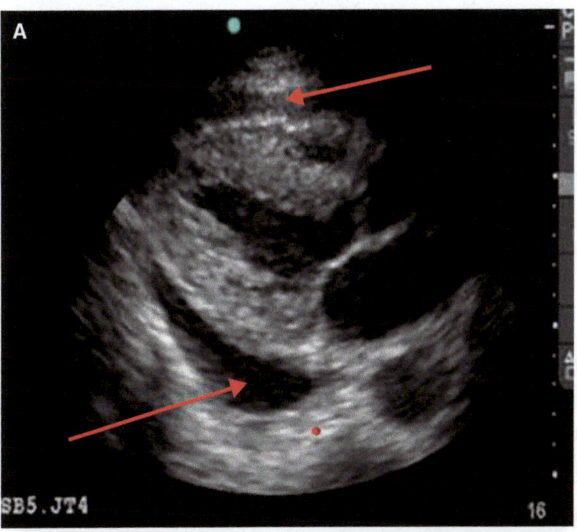


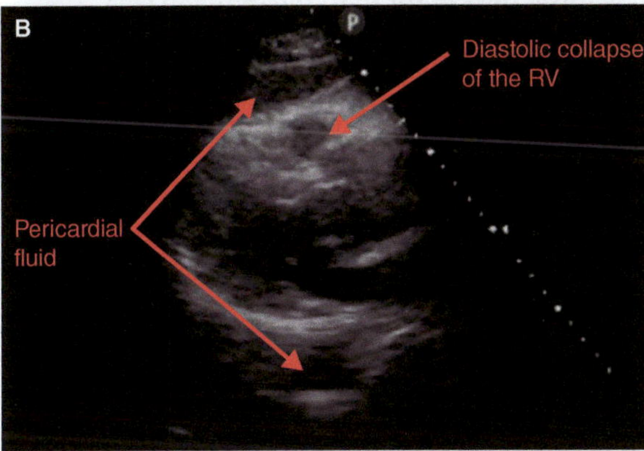


**Figure 6.2.** (A) Parasternal long axis with evidence of pericardial effusion (red arrows). Note non-cardiac preset. (B) Pericardial tamponade with large pericardial effusion and completely collapsible right ventricle. Note cardiac preset.

*Source:* Avila, M. (2019). Basic transthoracic echocardiography (cardiac ultrasound)—TTE made simple. POCUS 101. Retrieved from https://www.youtube.com/watch?v=1E4NSR6yjMw

- Subxiphoid/subcostal
  - Place probe below xiphoid process with marker facing patient's right
  - Angle probe superiorly toward left shoulder and apply gentle downward pressure on probe tip

> **PRO TIPS**
>
> A deep breath brings the heart downward into view.
>
> Ask the patient to bend knees to relax the abdominal muscles.

- Inferior vena cava (IVC)
  - Short axis
  - From the subcostal window angle, beam down.
  - The right atrium will lead to the IVC.
- Long axis
  - Rotate probe clockwise 90° (marker toward the patient's head)
  - Ensure hepatic vein connects to the IVC
  - Be aware, both the IVC and aorta can be pulsatile at this level and color doppler is helpful to aid in vessel delineation

## INTERPRETATION

**■ Pericardial effusion**

- Pericardial effusion often appears as anechoic/hypoechoic fluid.
- Pleural effusions will accumulate below the descending aorta while pericardial effusions will accumulate between the heart and the descending aorta in PLAX.

**Cardiac tamponade physiology**

- Rate of fluid accumulation is more important than the effusion size
  - Rapidly accumulating effusions can cause tamponade with as little as 150 to 250 mL, whereas chronic effusions (>1,000 mL) may not impair hemodynamics.
- Right atrial collapse (during ventricular systole) and/or RV collapse (during ventricular diastole) are concerning for tamponade physiology.
- A non-plethoric IVC (<2.1 cm) with >50% respiratory variation has a high negative predictive value favoring against tamponade (95%–97% sensitivity)[5]

**■ LV systolic function**

- Visual estimation
  - If the ventricular walls and the mitral valve barely move during systole, this is likely reduced EF.

**E-point septal separation (EPSS)**

- Estimates LVEF
- In PLAX, place M-mode cursor through tip of anterior mitral valve leaflet

- ○ Measure distance between valve and septum when valve is closest to the septum
- ○ Normal EPSS <0.7 cm
- ○ EPSS not accurate in aortic regurgitation or mitral valve stenosis.

- **Right heart strain**
  - Right heart strain, in the correct clinical situation, is indicative of pulmonary embolism; however, it is neither sensitive nor specific enough to rule out or rule in by ultrasound alone.
  - In A4C, is the RV larger than the LV?
    - ○ Normal RV:LV ratio is 0.6:1
  - In the PSSA view, does the LV appear like an O or D?
    - ○ A normal LV should appear like an O
    - ○ Right heart strain can cause septal flattening and make the LV look like the letter "D"
  - In PLAX, when RV appears larger than the aorta and right atrium, suspect right heart strain.
  - Tricuspid annular plane systolic excursion (TAPSE)
    - ○ In the A4C view, place M-mode cursor and measure movement of lateral tricuspid annulus
    - ○ <1.6 cm of movement between diastole and systole indicates RV systolic dysfunction

See Figure 6.3 for an image depicting right heart strain.

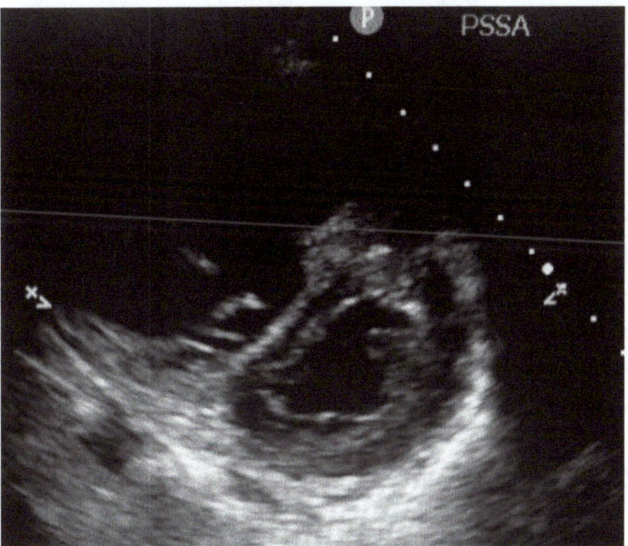


**Figure 6.3.** Right heart strain also known as "D-sign" demonstrates right ventricle wall collapse.

*Source:* Dihn, V. (n.d.). The D-Sign—Right heart strain from pressure v. volume overload. POCUS 101. Retrieved from https://www.pocus101.com/the-d-sign-right-heart-strain-from-pressure-vs-volume-overload/

■ **Volume responsiveness**
  - At the extremes and in conjunction with a clinical assessment, the IVC can be helpful in measuring volume responsiveness
  - IVC measurement guidelines
    ◦ IVC <2.1 cm + >50% collapse → Volume responsive (needs fluids)
    ◦ IVC >2.1 cm + <50% collapse → Suggests high right atrial pressure (e.g., congestive heart failure, tamponade)

See Table 6.3 for a summary of pathologic findings.

**Table 6.3** Summary of Pathologic Findings

| Condition | Findings |
|---|---|
| Reduced EF | Normal EF: >50%<br>Mild dysfunction: 40%–50%<br>Moderate dysfunction: 30%–40%<br>Severe dysfunction: <30%<br>EPSS >0.7 cm = reduced EF |
| Pericardial effusion/tamponade physiology | Rate of accumulation is more important than size of effusion in considering cardiac tamponade<br>Look for RV and/or right atrial collapse when each chamber should be filling<br>IVC <2.1 cm with >50% respiratory variation is unlikely tamponade physiology |
| Right heart strain | RV>LV in A4C<br>"D" sign in PSSA |
| Fluid status | IVC can be helpful at extremes, but use caution and consider other clinical parameters |

EF, ejection fraction; EPSS, E-point septal separation; IVC, Inferior vena cava; LV, left ventricular; PSSA, parasternal short axis; RV, right ventricular.

## PEARLS AND PITFALLS

■ If poor cardiac windows, consider alternative views
  - PLAX → Use left lateral decubitus position.
  - A4C → Have patient exhale fully and hold breath.
  - Subxiphoid → Have patient bend knees to relax abdominal wall.

■ In chronic lung disease, the heart may be significantly lower, making PLAX and PSSA views more difficult to obtain.

■ Consider rotating patients on their left side to obtain better windows; PSSA at the papillary level is the best window to visually estimate EF.

■ PSSA at mitral valve level will likely underestimate EF; PSSA at apex level will likely overestimate EF.

■ Rate of pericardial effusion accumulation is more important than size of effusion

■ Cardiac tamponade is a clinical diagnosis that can be aided by ultrasound.

■ In PLAX, be careful not to mistake a pleural effusion as a pericardial effusion.

- RV dilation alone does not confirm pulmonary embolism—consider chronic causes like chronic obstructive pulmonary disease, pulmonary hypertension, or left heart disease.
- A flipped probe marker in A4C will flip LV/RV on screen.
- Moderator band is in RV

## VIDEOS

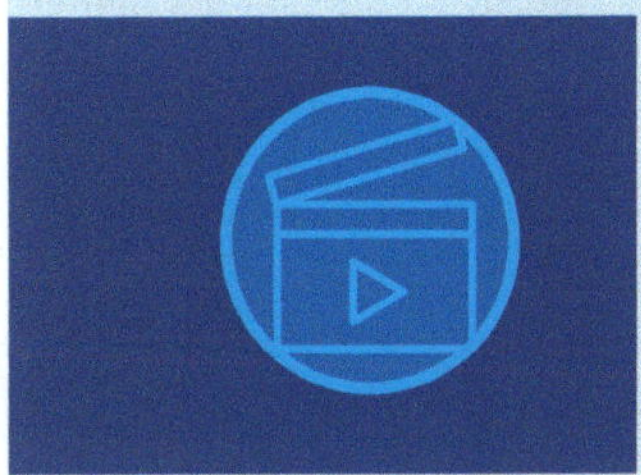

- Cardiac Introduction
- Estimating Ejection Fraction
- Parasternal Long Axis
- Parasternal Short Axis
- Pericardial Effusion
- Right Ventricle Function
- Subxiphoid/Subcostal View

**To access the videos, please go to the List of Videos in the front matter.**

## BIBLIOGRAPHY


Alerhand, S., & Carter, J. M. (2019). What echocardiographic findings suggest a pericardial effusion is causing tamponade? *American Journal of Emergency Medicine, 37*(2), 321–326. https://doi.org/10.1016/j.ajem.2018.11.004

American College of Emergency Physicians (2006). Emergency ultrasound imaging criteria compendium. American College of Emergency Physicians. *Annals of emergency medicine, 48*(4), 487–510. https://doi.org/10.1016/j.annemergmed.2006.07.946

Dresden, S., Mitchell, P., Rahimi, L., Leo, M., Rubin-Smith, J., Bibi, S., White, L., Langlois, B., Sullivan, A., & Carmody, K. (2014). Right ventricular dilatation on bedside echocardiography performed by emergency physicians aids in the diagnosis of pulmonary embolism. *Annals of Emergency Medicine, 63*(1), 16–24. https://doi.org/10.1016/j.annemergmed.2013.08.016

Klein, A. L., Abbara, S., Agler, D. A., Appleton, C. P., Asher, C. R., Hoit, B., Hung, J., Garcia, M. J., Kronzon, I., Oh, J. K., Rodriguez, E. R., Schaff, H. V., Schoenhagen, P., Tan, C. D., & White, R. D. (2013). American Society of Echocardiography clinical recommendations for multimodality cardiovascular imaging of patients with pericardial disease: Endorsed by the Society for Cardiovascular Magnetic Resonance and Society of Cardiovascular Computed Tomography. *Journal of the American Society of Echocardiography, 26*(9), 965–1012.e15. https://doi.org/10.1016/j.echo.2013.06.023

Mandavia, D. P., Hoffner, R. J., Mahaney, K., & Henderson, S. O. (2001). Bedside echocardiography by emergency physicians. *Annals of Emergency Medicine, 38*(4), 377–382. https://doi.org/10.1067/mem.2001.118224

Moore, C. L., Rose, G. A., Tayal, V. S., Sullivan, D. M., Arrowood, J. A., & Kline, J. A. (2002). Determination of left ventricular function by emergency physician echocardiography of hypotensive patients. *Academic Emergency Medicine, Official Journal of the Society for Academic Emergency Medicine, 9*(3), 186–193. https://doi.org/10.1111/j.1553-2712.2002.tb00242.x

# CHAPTER 7

# GALLBLADDER ULTRASOUND

Christopher Deonarine

## INTRODUCTION

- Eight percent of men and 17% of women will suffer from gallbladder disease, which is the third leading cause of abdominal pain presentation (American College of Emergency Physicians [ACEP], 2025).
- Point-of-care ultrasound (POCUS) provides a rapid, noninvasive method to evaluate gallbladder pathology and identification of cholelithiasis by novice scanners with sensitivity and specificity of 86% and 88% (ACEP, 2025).
- Five hallmark findings of cholecystitis include wall thickness, presence of gallstones, sonographic Murphy's sign, pericholecystic fluid and common bile duct (CBD) measurements which are all identifiable with POCUS, reducing time to diagnosis and intervention (ACEP, 2025).
- Absence of gallstones has a 100% negative predictive value (Villar et al., 2015).
- Cholelithiasis with positive sonographic Murphy's sign has a 90% positive predictive value (Villar et al., 2015)

See Tables 7.1 and 7.2 for indications and differentials.

**Table 7.1** Indications

| RUQ pain | Nausea, vomiting, diarrhea, fever | Epigastric pain |
|---|---|---|
| Chest pain, pleuritic pain | Flank pain, trauma | Peritonitis |

RUQ, right upper quadrant.

**Table 7.2** Differentials

| Cholecystitis, Cholelithiasis | Colangitis, Choledocolithiasis | Peptic ulcer disease, GERD | Pulmonary infection | Right nephrolithiasis or pyelonephritis |
|---|---|---|---|---|
| Liver cirrhosis, mass, abscess, tumor, ascites | Pancreatitis, pancreatic mass | Gastritis | AAA | ACS |

AAA, abdominal aortic aneurysm; ACS, acute coronary syndrome; GERD, gastroesophageal reflux disease.

## IMAGE ACQUISITION

- **Probe:** Curvilinear

> **PRO TIP**
>
> Change to the phased array to obtain intercostal images.

- **Preset:** gallbladder, abdomen, or Focused Assessment with Sonography in Trauma (FAST)
- **Hand placement:** Hold the transducer like a pencil.
- **Technique**
  - Patient position: Supine initially, left lateral decubitus is helpful to bring the gallbladder closer to the probe.
  - Scanner position: Stand on the patient's right side.
  - Initially probe should be in long axis with probe marker cephalad below the right costal margin in the midclavicular line.
  - Gently apply pressure, slide laterally and tilt the probe further cephalad into the subcostal margin.
  - Angle the transducer slightly toward the patient's right shoulder if needed.

> **PRO TIP**
>
> Remember the gallbladder can be found in many different anatomical locations.

  - Short access view of the gallbladder—simply rotate the transducer 90° with the indicator pointing toward scanner's left
  - Scanner may also start in midline in short access view, sliding with gentle pressure to the scanner's left until the gallbladder comes into view in its circular/oblong shape, anechoic in appearance with hyperechoic defined walls.
  - Scanner may also scan starting in midclavicular position, tilting/fanning the probe to acquire proper view of the gallbladder.
  - Scanner may also have patient in a modified left lateral decubitus position and scan from the posterior aspect near posterior midaxillary line.

## IMAGE INTERPRETATION

- **Long axis view**
  - Gallbladder, inferior vena cava, and portal vein (PV) should be visible
  - Gallbladder is an elongated, hypoechoic, and oblong structure
  - Portal triad evaluation demonstrates the classic "Mickey Mouse" sign
    - Portal vein, CBD, and hepatic artery (HA)
    - All structures will present hypoechoic

> **PRO TIP**
>
> CBD should be measured from inner wall to inner wall in the longitudinal plane using color Doppler to differentiate it from the HA and PV.

- CBD diameter
  - <6 mm (normal in young adults)
  - 6 to 8 mm (borderline dilation, consider age and postcholecystectomy status)
  - >8 mm (concerning for obstruction, evaluate for choledocholithiasis or biliary stricture)
- Cholelithiasis appears as hyperechoic structures with posterior acoustic shadowing.
- Sludge: hyperechoic, no shadowing, may layer dependently
- Polyps: hyperechoic, no shadowing, typically immobile

■ **Short axis view**

- Gallbladder and duodenum often visible
- Gallbladder is hypoechoic and circular in shape

**PRO TIP**

Excellent view for measuring wall thickness and presence of pericholecystic fluid.

■ Gallbladder wall
  - Normal <4 mm
■ Pericholecystic fluid
  - anechoic presentation surrounding or adjacent to gallbladder wall

## ANATOMY/IMAGES

See Figure 7. 1 Normal gallbladder anatomy in longitudinal view. Figure 7. 2 Normal gallbladder anatomy in transverse view.

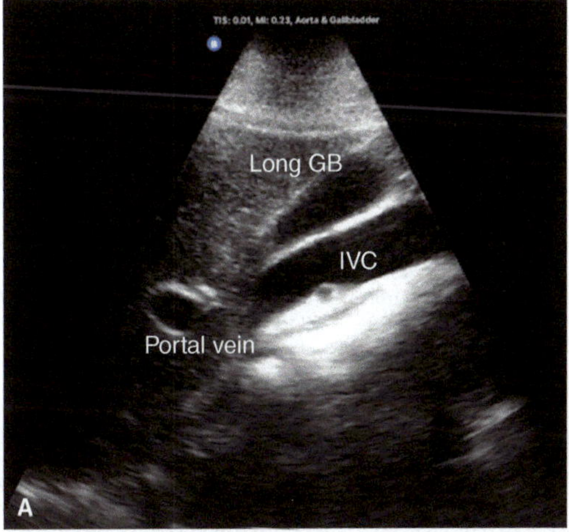


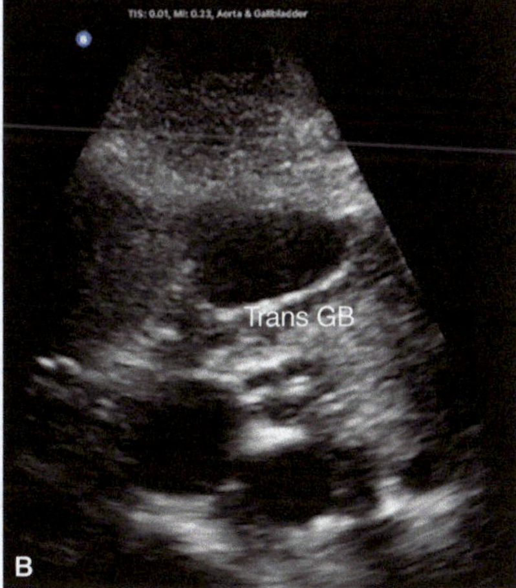


**Figure 7.1.** Normal gallbladder (GB) anatomy. (A) Longitudinal GB. (B) Transverse GB.
*Source:* Used with permission. Image courtesy of Dr. Kelli Craven.

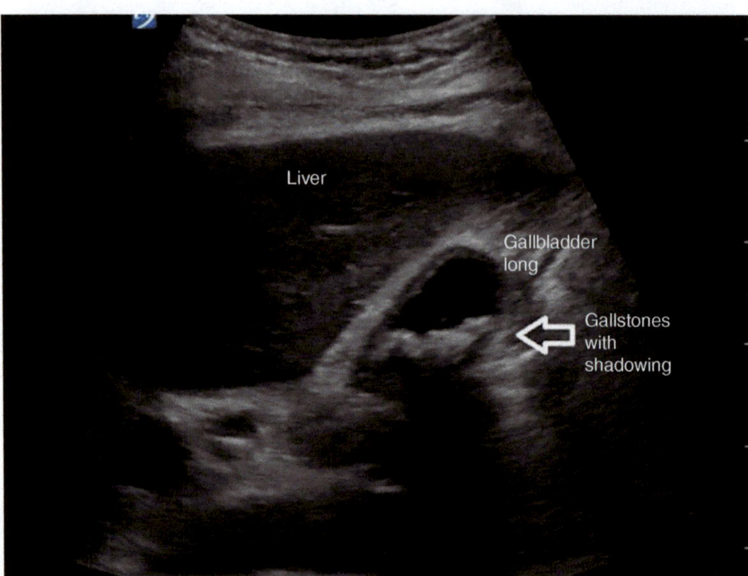


**Figure 7.2.** Gallbladder point-of-care ultrasound concerning for acute cholecystitis with gallbladder with thickened anterior wall and shadowing gallstones.
*Source*: Yang, F. J., Kohen, B., Sanapala, S., & Halperin, M. (2022). A potential pitfall in POCUS of the gallbladder: Beware of the duodenum. *POCUS Journal, 7*(2), 188–189. https://doi.org/10.24908/pocus.v7i2.15632

See Table 7.3 for a summary of pathologic findings.

**Table 7.3** Summary of Pathologic Findings

| Ultrasound (US) Finding | Normal Gallbladder | Acute Cholecystitis |
|---|---|---|
| US + Murphy's sign | Absent | Present |
| Gallbladder content | Anechoic | Stones (hyperechoic with shadowing), sludge/pus (isoechoic) |
| Wall edema | Absent | Present |
| Diffuse wall thickness | Absent | Present |
| Transverse diameter | <4 cm | >4 cm |
| Longitudinal diameter | <8 cam | >8 cm |
| Pericholecystic fluid | Absent | Present (anechoic free fluid) |

## PEARLS AND PITFALLS

- Ask the patient to take a deep breath or have the patient lie in the left lateral decubitus position.
- Bowel gas obstructing views—apply gentle pressure to displace the bowel gas and allow visualization of the gallbladder.

■ A contracted gallbladder post-meal may be misinterpreted as thickened wall or sludge—ideally, scan patients after at least 6 hours of fasting.

■ Tumefactive sludge does not produce shadowing and should not be confused for cholelithiasis

■ Ensure posterior acoustic enhancement or edge artifact is not mistaken for pericholecystic fluid. True fluid collections will be anechoic and surround the gallbladder.

■ Do not confuse ascites with pericholecystic fluid

## BIBLIOGRAPHY

American College of Emergency Physicians. (2009). Emergency ultrasound guidelines. *Annals of Emergency Medicine, 53*(4), 550–570. https://doi.org/10.1016/j.annemergmed.2008.12.013

American College of Emergency Physicians. (2020). *Sonoguide basics: Gallbladder*. Retrieved April 2, 2025, from https://www.acep.org/sonoguide/basic/gallbladder

Dumbrava, B. D., Bass, G. A., Jumean, A., Birido, N., Corbally, M., Pereira, J., Biloslavo, A., Zago, M., & Walsh, T. N. (2023). The accuracy of point-of-care ultrasound (POCUS) in acute gallbladder disease. *Diagnostics (Basel, Switzerland), 13*(7), 1248. https://doi.org/10.3390/diagnostics13071248

Jones, M. W., Genova, R., & O'Rourke, M. C. (2023). Acute cholecystitis. In *StatPearls* [Internet]. StatPearls Publishing. Retrieved April 2, 2025, from https://www.ncbi.nlm.nih.gov/books/NBK459171/

Soni, N. J., Arntfield, R., & Kory, P. (2020). *Point of care ultrasound* (2nd ed.). Elsevier.

Villar, J., Summers, S. M., Menchine, M. D., Fox, J. C., & Wang, R. (2015). The absence of gallstones on Point-of-Care Ultrasound rules out acute cholecystitis. *Journal of Emergency Medicine, 49*(4), 475–480. https://doi.org/10.1016/j.jemermed.2015.04.037

Zenobii, M. F., Accogli, E., Domanico, A., & Arienti, V. (2016). Update on bedside ultrasound (US) diagnosis of acute cholecystitis (AC). *Intern in Emergency Medicine, 11*, 261–264. https://doi.org/10.1007/s11739-015-1342-1

# CHAPTER 8

# RENAL ULTRASOUND

Christopher Deonarine

## INTRODUCTION

- Point-of-care ultrasound (POCUS) is a rapid, radiation-free tool for assessing renal pathology, including hydronephrosis and nephrolithiasis in patients with flank pain, hematuria, or dysuria.
- POCUS has high sensitivity (72%–97%) and specificity (73%–98%) for diagnosing hydronephrosis, reducing the need for CT in select patients.

See Tables 8.1 and 8.2.

**Table 8.1** Indications

| Flank pain, back pain | Dysuria, urgency, frequency | Hematuria, oliguria |
|---|---|---|
| Trauma | Fever, hemodynamic instability | Dialysis, abnormal labs |

**Table 8.2** Differentials

| Nephrolithiasis, Hydronephrosis | AAA, ACS, Pulmonary infection | Renal cyst, mass |
|---|---|---|
| Bladder outlet obstruction | CKD | Trauma |

AAA, abdominal aortic aneurysm; ACS, acute coronary syndrome; CKD, chronic kidney disease.

## IMAGE ACQUISITION

- **Probe:** curvilinear
- **Preset:** abdomen, renal
- **Hand placement**
  - Renal assessment—cup the transducer in the palm
  - Bladder assessment—hold like a pencil
- **Technique**
  - Patient positioning: supine
  - Always maintain proper position of probe marker to determine proper planes and anatomical position.

- Renal windows best obtained with probe marker toward the head
- Left kidney best visualized along the posterior axillary line with "knuckles to the bed and probe pointing toward the head"
- Right kidney is best seen along the midaxillary line at the most inferior intercostal space.

## ANATOMY/IMAGES

See Figure 8.1 for normal right renal appearance.

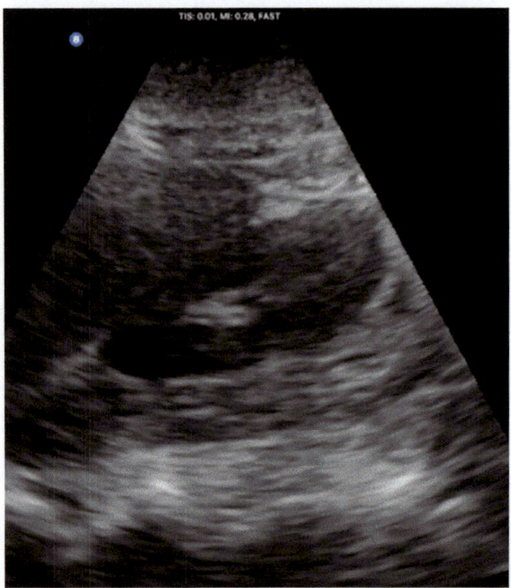

**Figure 8.1.** Normal right renal appearance.
*Source:* Used with permission. Image courtesy of Dr. Kelli Craven.

## INTERPRETATION

- **Normal renal anatomy**
  - Length: 9 to 12 cm
  - Width: 4 to 6 cm
  - Cortical thickness: ≥1 cm
  - Cortex = echogenic
  - Medulla = anechoic
- **Mild hydronephrosis:** separation of renal sinus, small calyceal dilation with preserved papillae
- **Moderate hydronephrosis:** blunting of calyces with progressive loss of papillary structure without affecting the cortical thickness

- **Severe Hydronephrosis:** marked calyceal dilation, cortical thinning, and possible renal atrophy
- Nephrolithiasis demonstrates a small hyperechoic circular image with posterior acoustic shadowing.
- When color Doppler is applied to the area of suspected nephrolithiasis, look for the "twinkle sign," which appears as a mix of red and blue color signals due to the turbulent sound associated with rough interfaces caused by vascular calcification or nephrolithiasis.

## PEARLS AND PITFALLS

- If the kidney is difficult to visualize, have the patient take a deep breath and hold it to displace the kidney inferiorly and anteriorly.
- Use color Doppler to distinguish between hydronephrosis (no flow) and dilated renal vessels (pulsatile flow).
- If you spot an area of concern for nephrolithiasis, apply color Doppler and observe for the "twinkle sign" to help support diagnosis.

### VIDEOS

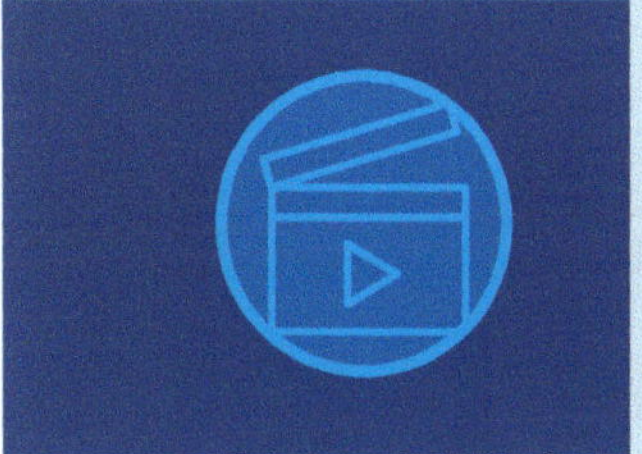

- Renal Ultrasound

**To access the videos, please go to the List of Videos in the front matter.**

## BIBLIOGRAPHY


Campbell, S. C., Cullinan, J. A., & Rubens, D. J. (2004). Slow flow or no flow? Color and power doppler us pitfalls in the abdomen and pelvis. *RadioGraphics, 24,* 497–506. https://doi.org/10.1148/rg .242035130

Coe, F. L., Evan, A., & Worcester, E. (2005). Kidney stone disease. *Journal of Clinical Investigation, 115*(10), 2598–2608. https://doi.org/10.1172/JCI26662

Einstein, A. J., Henzlova, M. J., & Rajagopalan, S. (2007). Estimating risk of cancer associated with radiation exposure from 64- slice computed tomography coronary angiography. *Journal of the American Medical Association, 298*(3), 317–323. https://doi.org/10.1001/jama.298.3.317

Gaspari, R. J., & Horst, K. (2005, December). Emergency ultrasound and urinalysis in the evaluation of flank pain. *Academic Emergency Medicine, 12*(12), 1180–1184. https://doi.org/10.1197/j.aem .2005.06.023

Jarrett, B. (n.d.). Renal/GU. The POCUS Atlas. https://www.thepocusatlas.com/renal-gu

Lanoix, R., Leak, L. V., Gaeta, T., & Gernsheimer, J. R. (2000). A preliminary evaluation of emergency ultrasound in the setting of an emergency medicine training program. *American Journal of Emergency Medicine, 18*(1), 41–45. https://doi.org/10.1016/S0735-6757(00)90046-9

Menon, M., Parulkar, B., & Darch, G. (1998). Urinary lithiasis: Etiology, diagnosis and medical management. In M. F. Campbell, P. C. Walsh, & A. B. Retik (Eds.), *Campbell's urology* (7th ed., pp. 2661–2733). Saunders.

Mitchell, D. G. (1990). Color doppler imaging: Principles, limitations, and artifacts. *Radiology, 177,* 1–10. https://doi.org/10.1148/radiology.177.1.2204956

Pathan, S. A, Mitra, B., Mirza, S., Momin, U., Ahmed, Z., Andraous, L. G., Shukla, D., Shariff, M. Y., Makki, M. M., George, T. T., Khan, S. S., Thomas, S. H., & Cameron, P. A. (2018, October). Emergency physician interpretation of point-of-care ultrasound for identifying and grading of hydronephrosis in renal colic compared with consensus interpretation by emergency radiologists. *Academic Emergency Medicine, 25*(10), 1129–1137. https://doi.org/10.1111/acem.13432

Singh, S. (n.d.). Renal/GU. The POCUS Atlas. https://www.thepocusatlas.com/renal-gu

Smith-Bindman, R., Aubin, C., Bailitz, J., Bengiamin, R. N., Camargo, C. A. Jr, Corbo, J., Dean, A. J., Goldstein, R. B., Griffey, R. T., Jay, G. D., Kang, T. L., Kriesel, D. R., Ma, O. J., Mallin, M., Manson, W., Melnikow, J., Miglioretti, D. L., Miller, S. K., Mills, L. D., … Cummings, S. R. (2014, September 18). Ultrasonography versus computed tomography for suspected nephrolithiasis. *New England Journal of Medicine, 371*(12), 1100–1110. https://doi.org/10.1056/NEJMoa1404446

Taus, P. J., Manivannan, S., & Dancel, R. (2022). Bedside assessment of the kidneys and bladder using point of care ultrasound. *POCUS Journal, 7*(2), 94–104. https://doi.org/10.24908/pocus.v7iKidney.15347

Vallone, G., Napolitano, G., Fonio, P., Antinolfi, G., Romeo, A., Macarini, L., Genovese, E. A., & Brunese, L. (2013). US detection of renal and ureteral calculi in patients with suspected renal colic. *Critical Ultrasound Journal, 5*(1), S3. https://doi.org/10.1186/2036-7902-5-S1-S3

Wong, C., Teitge, B., Ross, M., Young, P., Robertson, H. L., & Lang, E. (2018, June). The accuracy and prognostic value of point-of-care ultrasound for nephrolithiasis in the emergency department: A systematic review and meta-analysis. *Academic Emergency Medicine, 25*(6), 684–698. https://doi.org/10.1111/acem.13388

# CHAPTER 9

# DEEP VEIN THROMBOSIS OF UPPER AND LOWER EXTREMITY

Meghan Petzy

## INTRODUCTION

- The annual incidence of deep vein thrombosis (DVT) in the U.S. is approximately 1.6 per 1,000 people, with 300,000 deaths annually attributed to pulmonary embolism (PE).
- Failing to diagnose DVT can lead to PE.
- PE originates from a lower extremity (LE) DVT in 70% to 90% of cases, making early identification critical.
- Death occurs in approximately 6% of DVTs and 12% of PEs within 1 month of diagnosis.
- Upper extremity (UE) DVT accounts for 10% to 30% of all DVT cases, with central venous catheters, pacemakers, and malignancy as key risk factors.
- Brief, focused training allows providers expedited assessment with high diagnostic accuracy in any clinical setting
  - LE DVT: 96% sensitivity, 97% specificity
  - UE DVT: 97% sensitivity, 96% specificity

See Tables 9.1 and 9.2.

**Table 9.1** Indications

| UE/LE unilateral pain, swelling, tenderness, erythema | Positive Homan's Sign | Immobility, recent fracture/trauma. +Wells Criteria | Dialysis catheter, previous CVC access, IVDU |
|---|---|---|---|
| Voice changes, neck discomfort | Chest pain, Dyspnea | Pregnancy | COVID-19 infection |

CVC, central venous catheter; IVDU, intravenous drug use; LE, lower extremity; UE, upper extremity.

**Table 9.2** Differentials

| Cellulitis, superficial thrombophlebitis | Contact dermatitis | Trauma, Fractures, Compression injury, Compartment syndrome | Venous insufficiency, varicose veins, Lymphangitis | Baker's cyst |
|---|---|---|---|---|
| Thoracic outlet syndrome, Lymphadenitis | Sickle cell crisis, chest syndrome | ACS, AAA | Heart failure | Thrombophilia, Coagulopathies, CA, blood dyscrasias |

AAA, abdominal aortic aneurysm; ACS, acute coronary syndrome; CA, cardiac arrest.

## IMAGE ACQUISITION

- **Probe:** linear
- **Patient position:** supine with affected leg externally rotated and slightly flexed at the knee
- **Scanner position:** on the affected side
- **Hand placement**
  - LE: Hold probe like a pencil, transverse view, probe marker to scanner's left
  - UE: Hold probe like a pencil, transverse view, probe marker to scanner's left

**PRO TIP**

Saphenous vein—scan in transverse and longitudinal with plane.

- **Technique**
  - Preset: vascular
  - Probe marker to scanner's left
  - Apply medium to firm pressure with the probe until the artery compresses slightly and the vein compresses completely while moving through the scanning positions.
  - Scan the entire femoral and popliteal vein course systematically.
  - A fully compressible vein rules out DVT. Inability to compress the vein is the primary diagnostic criterion for DVT.

See Table 9.3 for LE scanning positions and Table 9.4 for UE scanning positions.

**Table 9.3** Lower Extremity Scanning Positions

| Femoral vein | Saphenofemoral junction | Bifurcation of common femoral vein | Deep femoral vein |
|---|---|---|---|
| Superficial femoral vein | Popliteal vein | Trifurcation of popliteal vein | Iliac veins (optional in cases of suspected proximal DVT) |

DVT, Deep vein thrombosis.

**Table 9.4** Upper Extremity Scanning Positions

| IJV | Subclavian vein | Axillary vein |
|---|---|---|
| Cephalic vein | Basilic vein | Brachial vein |

IJV, internal jugular vein.

**PRO-TIP**

While there is no strong evidence that compression ultrasound causes PE, avoid excessive compression if DVT is suspected.

## ANATOMY/IMAGES

See Figures 9.1 and 9.2 demonstrate normal images of common femoral vein and artery with color flow Doppler, and pathologic findings of deep vein thrombus appearance.

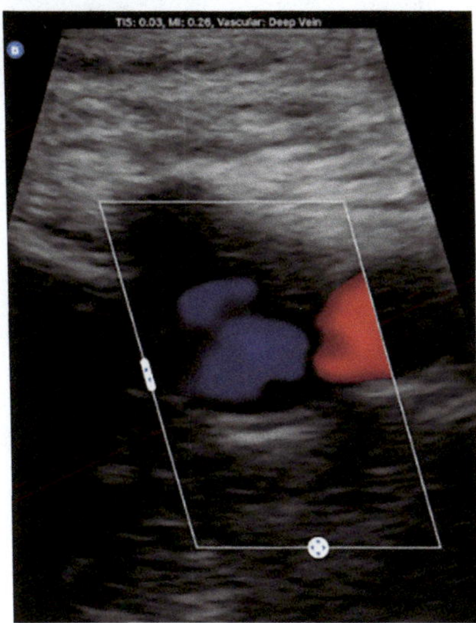

**Figure 9.1.** Common femoral vein and artery with color flow Doppler.

*Source:* Used with permission. Image courtesy of Dr. Kelli Craven.

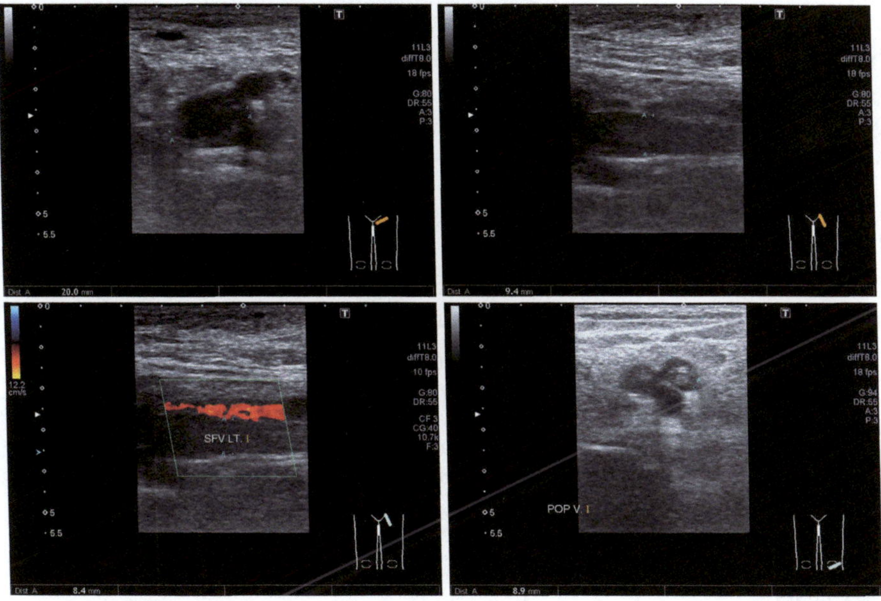

**Figure 9.2.** Hyperechoic thrombus with dilation of veins, at left superficial femoral vein and popliteal vein in both transverse and longitudinal views. Impression: Acute deep vein thrombosis (DVT) of left leg.

*Source:* Rattanachot2525/Dreamstime.com

## INTERPRETATION

- **Acute DVT:**
  - Anechoic or hypoechoic clot
  - Loosely adherent to vessel wall
  - Incomplete vein compression on ultrasound
- Chronic DVT:
  - Echogenic clot with increased fibrosis
  - Firmly attached to vessel wall
  - May not completely obstruct flow

See Table 9.5 for a summary of pathologic findings.

**Table 9.5** Summary of Pathologic Findings

| Condition | Ultrasound Findings |
|---|---|
| Deep vein thrombosis | Lack of compressibility, direct visualization, filling defect with color flow Doppler |
| Acute—direct visualization | Anechoic or hypoechoic, loosely attached to the vessel wall |
| Subacute or chronic—direct visualization | Echogenic, often visualized without compression, firmly attached to the vessel wall |

## PEARLS AND PITFALLS

- Appearance of thrombi can vary based on age, extent, and location.
- Incomplete compression of a vein is the main diagnostic criterion for DVT, even if the thrombus is not visualized.
- Ensure compression is applied only in the transverse plane, as longitudinal scanning does not confirm compressibility.
- Compare to contralateral side
- Apply gel down the extremity before scanning to maintain skin contact and sliding of probe.
- Normal venous valves may appear as echogenic structures, but they should move freely and not cause luminal obstruction.
- Color flow Doppler can aid in distinguishing vessels from other structures.
- Femoral vein = superficial femoral vein. HOWEVER, it is considered a deep vein
- Acute versus chronic DVT: residual thrombosis may be present indefinitely and with various echogenicity, acute often has a hyperechoic wall
- Technically limited studies
  - LE: obesity, edema, recent surgery or trauma, skin lesions, contractures, or leg casts
  - UE: presence of venous catheters, ports, pacemakers, automatic implantable cardioverter-defibrillators (AICDs), fistulas
- DVT mimics: lymph nodes, Baker's cyst, pseudoaneurysm ("yin/yang" sign), superficial thrombophlebitis, groin hematoma

## BIBLIOGRAPHY


Bauer, K., & Huismen, M. (2022, October 25). Clinical presentation and diagnosis of the nonpregnant adult with suspected deep vein thrombosis of the lower extremity. *UpToDate*. Retrieved January 12, 2024, from https://www.uptodate.com/contents/clinical-presentation-and-diagnosis-of-the-nonpregnant-adult-with-suspected-deep-vein-thrombosis-of-the-lower-extremity

Cuker, A., & Peyvandi, F. (2024, January 31). COVID-19: Hypercoagulability. UpToDate. Retrieved February 14, 2024, from https://www.uptodate.com/contents/covid-19-hypercoagulability

Dinh, V. (2023.). Ultrasound machine basics-knobology, probes, and modes. *POCUS 101*. https://www.pocus101.com/ultrasound-machine-basics-knobology-probes-and-modes/

Dinh, V., & Ahn, J. (2023). DVT ultrasound made easy: Step-by-step guide. *POCUS 101*. https://www.pocus101.com/dvt-ultrasound-made-easy-step-by-step-guide/

Eisner, D. (2023). Cost-effective management of deep-vein thrombosis. *Journal of Urgent Care Medicine, 37–39*. https://www.jucm.com/wp-content/uploads/2023/02/2022-17437-39-Case-Report.pdf

Khan, M. S., Sabnis, V. B., Phansalkar, D. S., Prasad, S. P., & Karnam, A. H. F. (2015). Use of ultrasound in peripheral venous catheterization in adult emergency and critical care units. *Anaesthesia Pain & Intensive Care, 19*(3), 303–310. https://www.apicareonline.com/index.php/APIC/article/view/360

Malhotra, A., & Lockwood, C. (2013). Deep vein thrombosis in pregnancy: Epidemiology, pathogenesis, and diagnosis. *UpToDate*. Retrieved January 12, 2024, from https://www.uptodate.com/contents/deep-vein-thrombosis-in-pregnancy-epidemiology-pathogenesis-and-diagnosis

Merschel, M. (2022, September 19). Blood clot risk remains elevated nearly a year after COVID-19. *American Heart Association*. https://www.heart.org/en/news/2022/09/19/blood-clot-risk-remains-elevated-nearly-a-year-after-covid-19

POCUS 101. (n.d.). *Complete ultrasound CPT codes list and reimbursement rates*. https://www.pocus101.com/complete-ultrasound-cpt-code-list-and-reimbursement-rates/

Pomero, F., Borretta, V., Bonzini, M., Melchio, R., Douketis, J. D., Fenoglio, L. M., & Dentali, F. (2013). Accuracy of emergency physician–performed ultrasonography in the diagnosis of deep-vein thrombosis. *Thrombosis and Haemostasis, 109*(01), 137–145. https://doi.org/10.1160/th12-07-0473

Ramsingh, D., & Gatling, J. (2018). Teaching point-of-care ultrasound (POCUS) to the perioperative physician. *Education in Anesthesia*, 131–150. https://doi.org/10.1017/9781316822548.013

Schafer, J., & Stickles, S. (2020, August 18). Deep vein thrombosis (DVT). Sonoguide: *Ultrasound*. https://www.acep.org/sonoguide/basic/dvt/

Soni, N. J., Arntfield, R., & Kory, P. (2020). *Point-of-care ultrasound* (2nd ed.). Elsevier.

Stephenson, T. (2022, August 8). *Case report: The woman with the swollen left arm*. https://www.acepnow.com/article/case-report-the-girl-with-the-swollen-left-arm/

Themes, U. (2020, October 20). Of ultrasound guidance. *Anesthesia Key: Fastest Anesthesia & Intensive Care & Emergency Medicine Insight Engine*. https://aneskey.com/of-ultrasound-guidance/

Varrias, D., Palaiodimos, L., Balasubramanian, P., Barrera, C., Nauka, P., Arfaras-Melainis, A., Zamora, C., Zavras, P., Napolitano, M., Gulani, P., Ntaios, G., Faillace, R., & Galen, B. (2021). The use of point-of-care ultrasound (POCUS) in the diagnosis of deep vein thrombosis. *Journal of Clinical Medicine, 10*(17), 3903. https://doi.org/10.3390/jcm10173903

Waheed, S. M. (2023, January 19). Deep vein thrombosis. In *StatPearls* [Internet]. StatPearls Publishing. https://www.ncbi.nlm.nih.gov/books/NBK507708

# CHAPTER 10

# LUNG ULTRASOUND EXAM

Meghan Petzy

## INTRODUCTION

- Point of care ultrasound (POCUS) evaluates most lung pathologies expeditiously.
- May reduce the need for radiation-exposing imaging
- 90% of lung pathology involves the pleural line (Dinh, n.d.).
- Assess pleural surfaces at multiple sites and also assess the alveoli and interstitium in real- time dynamic imaging.
- Safe, validated, highly sensitive, and specific differentiation of the causes of respiratory failure
- POCUS supersedes physical exam and chest x-ray alone
- Lung ultrasound provides real-time dynamic imaging and can detect pneumothorax, pleural effusions, and interstitial syndromes with near-CT accuracy.
- Increasing use in acutely ill pediatric patients where avoiding radiation from x-rays or CT scans is a priority

See Tables 10.1 and 10.2 for indications and differentials.

**Table 10.1** Indications

| Chest pain | Dyspnea Tachypnea | Trauma | Hypoxia Hypoxemia | Wheezing |
|---|---|---|---|---|
| Signs of infection | Cough | Respiratory distress | Cancer or blood dyscrasias | Drug use, vaping, tobacco use |

**Table 10.2** Differentials

| Pneumonia | Pulmonary edema, effusion | ARDS COVID–19 Atelectasis | Pneumothorax Hemothorax | PE |
|---|---|---|---|---|
| Bronchiolitis, Bronchitis | Reactive airway disease | COPD Emphysema | Heart failure ACS | Mass mets TB Abscess Empyema |

ACS, acute coronary syndrome; ARDS, adult respiratory distress syndrome; COPD, chronic obstructive pulmonary disease; PE, pulmonary embolism; TB, tuberculosis.

## IMAGE ACQUISITION

- **Probe**
  - Phased array and curvilinear are ideal for deeper lung evaluation, including pleural effusion and consolidation.
  - Linear is optimal for pneumothorax detection given its superior resolution of the pleural line.
- **Patient position**
  - Anterior lung scanning: supine or sitting up, arm placed behind head for rib space access
  - Lateral lung scanning: sitting or lateral decubitus, arm raised to expose axillary region
  - Posterior lung scanning: sitting upright, arms crossed over chest to open rib spaces
- **Hand placement**
  - Hold like a pencil
- **Pediatrics**
- **Probe:** linear, curvilinear, or phased array
- **Patient position:** sitting in caregiver's lap, hugging the child for lateral and posterior images
- **Hand placement**
  - Hold like a pencil
- **Preset:**
  - Lung or abdominal

**PRO TIPS**

Turning off the lung preset may improve visualization of lung artifacts.

Pleural effusions may be better visualized using a cardiac preset.

  - Probe marker to scanner's left
  - Pleural line: 5 mm deep to the ribs, pleura: depth 7.5 to 10 cm
  - Lung parenchyma/lower lung fields: 13 to 16 cm

## SIX-POINT LUNG EXAM

- **Anterior chest:** points 1 and 2
  - Probe at the midclavicular line, second intercostal space
    - Identify two rib shadows = "batwing sign" (normal finding)
    - Posterior acoustic shadowing = wings
    - Hyperechoic pleural line = belly
    - Observe lung sliding = "ants marching"
      - Confirm lung sliding in M-mode = "seashore sign"

- ○ Observe for B-lines and A-lines
    - – B-lines ("lung rockets") run vertical
    - – A-lines are hyperechoic horizontal lines running parallel
- **Lateral chest:** points 3 and 4
  - Probe at right and left midaxillary line around sixth to seventh intercostal space
  - Observe for abnormal and normal findings
- **Posterior chest:** points 5 and 6
  - Posterolateral alveolar and/or pleural syndrome (PLAPS)
  - Assess for pleural effusion and consolidation
  - Indicator toward the patient's head
  - PLAPS point: intersection of posterior axillary line and a rib space between the 10th and 12th ribs
  - Identify the liver (on the right) or spleen (on the left), kidney, and diaphragm.
  - Find the spine: extends up until the border of the diaphragm and should stop
  - "Curtain sign"
    - ○ Normal at PLAPS position
    - ○ Appears like a "curtain" sweeping over organs during inhalation, organs reappear during exhalation
    - ○ Mirror image artifacts: reflection from a structure creates a false image

## IMAGE INTERPRETATION

- **B-lines**
  - Ray-like, hyperechoic vertical lines extending from pleural line, move with lung sliding

### PRO TIP

The presence of ≥3 B-lines per intercostal space suggests interstitial syndrome (e.g., pulmonary edema, adult respiratory distress syndrome [ARDS], pneumonia).

  - Bilateral B-lines = pulmonary edema, ARDS, interstitial lung disease
  - Unilateral B-lines = pneumonia, atelectasis, lung contusion, infarct, malignancy
- **Jellyfish sign**
  - Movement of lung tissue in pleural fluid = pleural effusion
- **Sinusoid sign**
  - Movement of floating lung toward and away from chest wall
  - Confirm in M-mode = free-flowing pleural fluid
- **Quad sign**
  - Pleural effusion with anechoic appearance, delineated by the pleural line, the rib shadows, and the lung line

- **Plankton sign**
  - Floating debris or bubbles swirling within fluid/loculations = parapneumonic effusion
- **Hematocrit sign**
  - Echogenic layering of material pleural effusion = exudative effusion or hemothorax
- **Hepatization of lung**
  - Well-defined lung parenchyma with similar echogenicity to the liver = consolidation
- **Shred sign**
  - Jagged edge within consolidated lobe = pneumonia
- **Air bronchograms**
  - Jagged border between consolidated and aerated lung = pneumonia
- **Spine sign**
  - Spine visualization past the diaphragm = consolidation or pleural effusion

## THE BLUE PROTOCOL

- Used in the diagnosis of acute respiratory failure
  - A-profile
    - A-lines + lung sliding → chronic obstructive pulmonary disease (COPD), pulmonary embolism (PE), pneumonia
  - A′-profile
    - A-lines + absent lung sliding → pneumothorax
  - B-profile
    - B-lines + lung sliding → pulmonary edema, interstitial syndrome
  - B′-profile
    - B-lines + absent lung sliding → pneumonia, ARDS
  - A/B profile:
    - One lung with A-lines, one with B-lines → pneumonia

## ANATOMY/IMAGES

See Figure 10.1 for normal lung finding, including the liver and diaphragm, Figure 10.2 for normal pleural line with A-lines (hyperechoic parallel lines), and Figure 10.3 for lung with lung sliding in M-Mode with evidence of lung pulse.

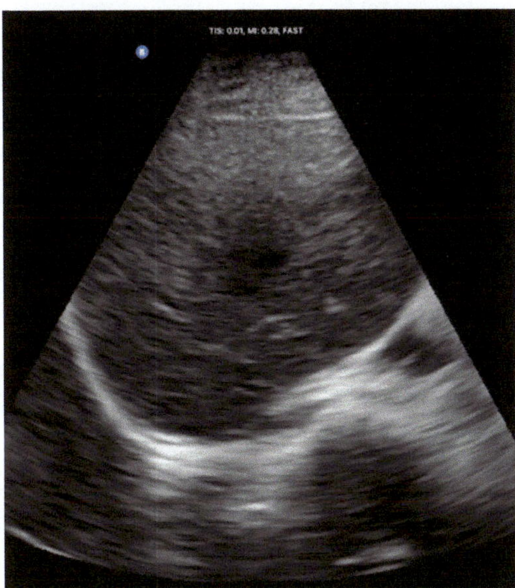

**Figure 10.1.** Normal lung finding—liver and diaphragm.
*Source:* Used with permission. Image courtesy of Dr. Kelli Craven.

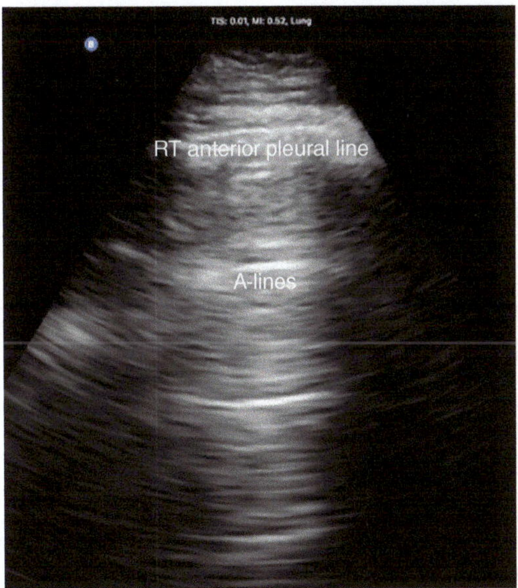


**Figure 10.2.** Normal pleural line with A-lines (hyperechoic parallel lines).
*Source:* Used with permission. Image courtesy of Dr. Kelli Craven.

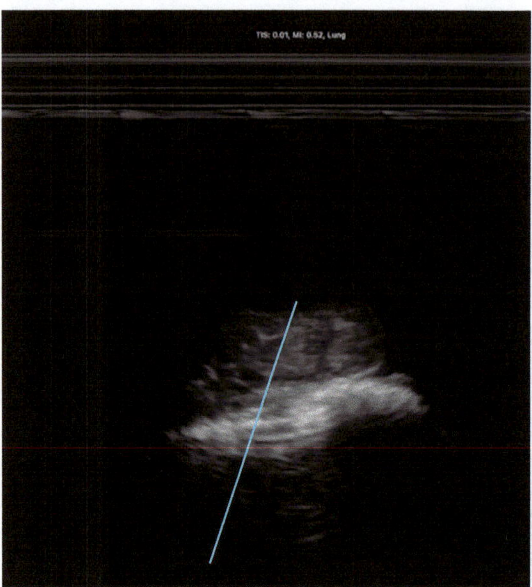


**Figure 10.3.** Lung with lung sliding in M-mode with evidence of lung pulse.

*Source:* Used with permission. Image courtesy of Dr. Kelli Craven.

See Table 10.3 for a summary of pathologic lung findings.

**Table 10.3** Summary of Pathologic Lung Findings

| Condition | Ultrasound Findings |
|---|---|
| Abscess/necrosis | Well-defined hypoechoic area within lobe |
| ARDS | Bilateral patchy B-lines, scattered A-lines, thickened pleural line |
| Atelectasis | Loss of lung volume, static air bronchograms |
| Bronchiolitis | B-lines in children less than 2 in winter months |
| COPD/asthma | Bilateral A-lines with normal lung sliding, reduced or absent lung sliding, no evidence of lung point |
| PE | Bilateral A-lines, right heart strain, + DVT |
| Metastatic lesions | Multiple varying echogenicities, invasion of chest wall/diaphragm, pleural effusion |
| COVID–19 | Separated B-lines, irregular pleural lines, confluent B-lines, bilateral consolidations, air bronchograms |
| Pleural effusionPulmonary edema | Anechoic area, spine, jellyfish, or sinusoid sign<br>Diffuse bilateral B-lines |
| Pneumonia | Focal unilateral B-lines, reduced lung sliding, lung hepatization sign, dynamic air bronchogram, shred or plankton sign |

ARDS, adult respiratory distress syndrome; COPD, chronic obstructive pulmonary disease; DVT, deep vein thrombosis; PE, pulmonary embolism.

## PEARLS AND PITFALLS

- When A- or B-lines are not visualized, reposition the probe between two ribs.
- Over gain images make it difficult to visualize A-lines.
- Body habitus may limit image quality.
- Ultrasound waves cannot pass through air if subcutaneous emphysema is present.
- Most lung pathology is not altered by patient position EXCEPT pleural effusions and interstitial syndromes.
- Patients with normal lung ultrasound + dyspnea = evaluate for COPD, asthma, PE, or other nonpulmonary pathologies
- A lung point (transition between lung sliding and absent sliding) is 100% specific for pneumothorax, but may not always be visible in large pneumothoraces.
- Lung sliding rules out a pneumothorax with 100% specificity.
- Absence of lung sliding alone is not diagnostic of pneumothorax—always correlate with M-mode (barcode sign) or the presence of a lung point.
- Absence of lung sliding can indicate other pathologies (pneumothorax, pleurodesis, decreased lung volume, reduced ventilation).
- Use color flow Doppler to differentiate between pleural masses, pleural effusions, and free-flowing fluid.
- COVID-19 pneumonia is characterized by irregular pleural lines, confluent B-lines, and bilateral subpleural consolidations, primarily affecting posterior lung fields.

## VIDEOS

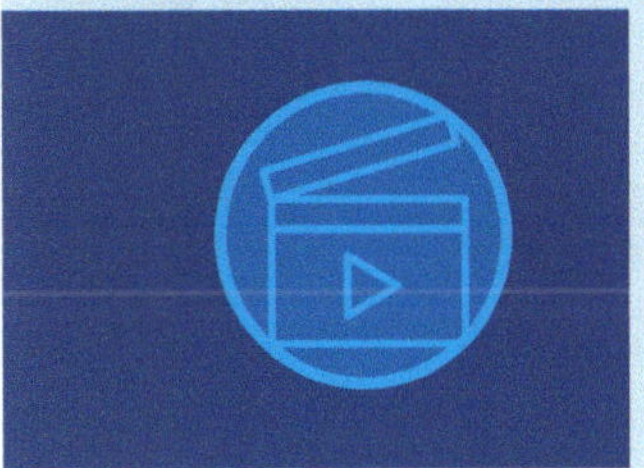

- Pleural Effusion—Thoracentesis
- Pleural Evaluation in Extended Focused Assessment With Sonography in Trauma (E-FAST) Exam

**To access the videos, please go to the List of Videos in the front matter.**

## BIBLIOGRAPHY

Dinh, V. (n.d.). Complete guide to lung ultrasound in covid-19 (coronavirus) patients. *POCUS 101*. https://www.pocus101.com/complete-guide-to-lung-ultrasound-in-covid-19-coronavirus-patients/

Dinh, V., & Deschamps, J. (n.d.). Lung ultrasound made easy: Step-by-step guide. *POCUS 101*. https://www.pocus101.com/lung-ultrasound-made-easy-step-by-step-guide/

Lichtenstein, D. A. (2014, January 9). Lung ultrasound in the critically ill. *Annals of Intensive Care, 4*(1), 1. https://doi.org/10.1186/2110-5820-4-1

Soni, N. J., Arntfield, R., & Kory, P. (2020). *Point of care ultrasound* (2nd ed.). Elsevier.

# CHAPTER 11

# OCULAR ULTRASOUND

Kelli Craven

## INTRODUCTION

- Safe non-ionizing radiation
- Resource-limited settings
- Real-time diagnosis for ophthalmologic emergencies at the bedside requiring immediate consultation and intervention
- Sensitivity 97% to 100%; specificity 83% to 97.2% (Soni et al., 2020)

See Tables 11.1 and 11.2 for indications and differentials.

**Table 11.1** Indications

| Eye pain | Red eye |
|---|---|
| Visual changes | Foreign body sensation |
| Orbital swelling | Trauma |

**Table 11.2** Differentials

| Globe rupture | Vitreous detachment Vitreous hemorrhage | Retinal detachment |
|---|---|---|
| Foreign body | Dislocated lens | Increased ICP |

ICP, intracranial pressure.

## IMAGE ACQUISITION

- **Probe**
  - Linear
- **Hand placement**
  - Hold the probe like a pencil or the "okay" sign.
- **Technique**
  - Place the small finger and ring finger on the bridge of the nose to stabilize the probe, which decreases probe pressure on the orbit.
  - Begin with a transverse scan (probe marker to the patient's right) to assess optic nerve sheath diameter (ONSD), then rotate 90°For a longitudinal view.

- Patient position: upright at 45°, position of comfort
- Scanner's position: side of scan with US in line of site
- Perform extraoccular movements intact (EOMI) in real-time with US visualization

**PRO TIP**

In a largely swollen eye unable to be opened, one can visualize the pupil response by having the patient look down; place the transducer on the bottom lid angled slightly cephalad, observe landmarks to identify the pupil, and shine light on the unaffected eye to observe for pupil response on the affected eye.

### ■ Equipment

- Ultrasound
- Linear probe
- Ultrasonic gel or gel pad
- Clear plastic adhesive cover (optional to cover the eye)
- Gloves
- Clean technique

## IMAGES

See Figures 11.1 through 11.3 for images depicting normal ocular anatomy and pathologic findings of ocular trauma to lens and hemorrhage.

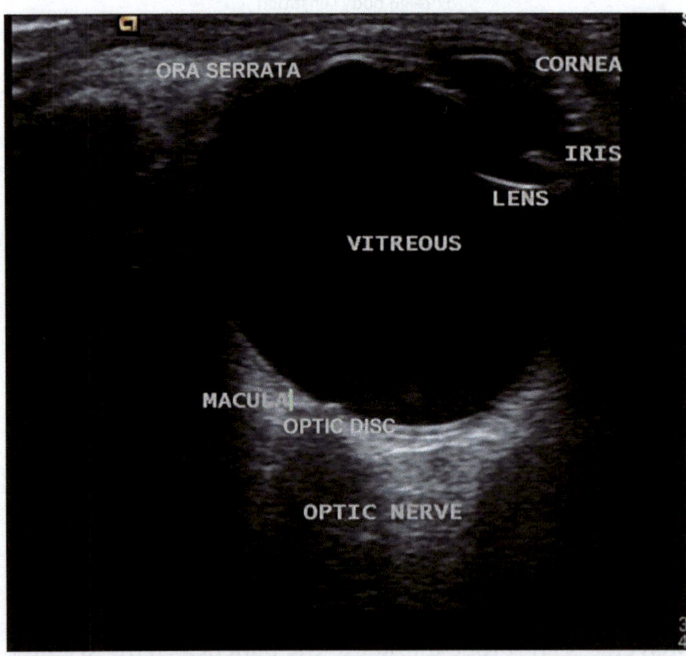


**Figure 11.1.** Normal ocular anatomy.

*Source:* Southern, S. (2009). Ultrasound of the eye. *Australasian Journal of Ultrasound in Medicine, 2*(1), 32–37. https://doi.org/10.1002/j.2205-0140.2009.tb00005.x

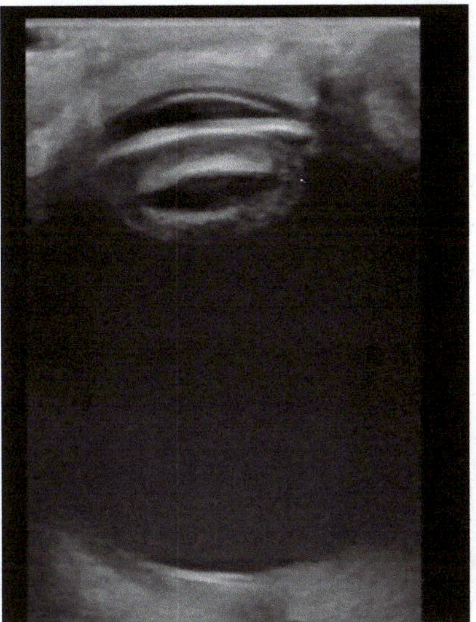

**Figure 11.2.** Ocular point-of-care ultrasound image of the patient's affected eye. Lens is irregular and thickened with increased echogenicity representative of traumatic cataract.

*Source:* Huffard, A., Overholt, S., Kantrales, A., & Hoffman, T. (2025). Acute traumatic cataract diagnosed by ocular point of care ultrasound (POCUS) in the emergency department. *POCUS Journal, 10*(1): 107–109. https://doi.org/10.24908/pocusj.v10i01.18110

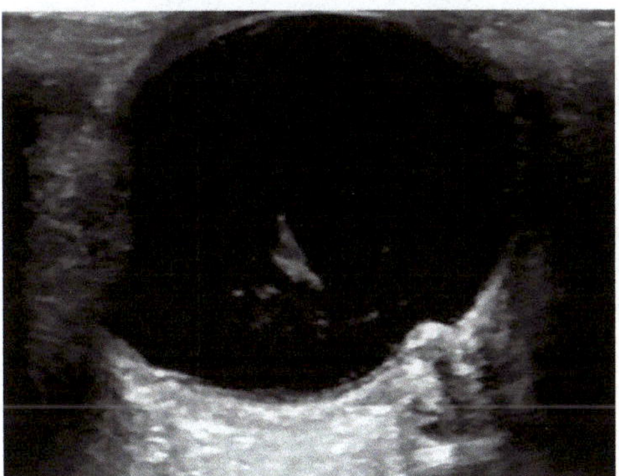

**Figure 11.3.** Hyperechoic debris in the vitreous chamber indicative of hemorrhage.

*Source:* Johnson, M. (2024). Terson syndrome diagnosed by ocular point of care ultrasound on the medical floor. *POCUS Journal, 9*(1): 36–40. https://doi.org/10.24908/pocus.v9i1.16660

## INTERPRETATION

- Any alteration in anatomic landmarks is likely pathology

**PRO TIP**

Be sure not to interpret air bubbles between clear film and eyelid as pathologic.

- The vitreous body should be hypoechoic without alterations in color and free of debris

- Optic nerve sheath diameter should be measured 8 to 10 mm from the globe or 3 mm behind the retina for the most accurate intracranial pressure (ICP) monitoring
  - <6 mm: normal ICP
  - ≥6 mm: strongly suggests intracranial hypertension (ICP >22 mmHg)
- There should be no evidence of papilledema as this indicates increased ICP

See Table 11.3 for a summary of pathologic findings.

**Table 11.3** Summary of Pathologic Findings

| Condition | Ultrasound Findings |
|---|---|
| Retinal detachment | Retina is completely detached from posterior aspect away from the optic nerve and appears as a thin, hyperechoic membrane tethered at the optic disc, often seen moving with eye motion. |
| Vitreous detachment | Retina remains attached at the pole near optic nerve. |
| Increased ICP | ICP >22 cause papilledema and increased ONSD |
| Globe rupture | Complete loss of all landmarks |
| Lens dislocation | Dislocated lens will maintain its shape even if displaced from normal anatomical landmark |
| Foreign body | Hyperechoic appearing object in any location |

ICP, intracranial pressure; ONSD, optic nerve sheath diameter.

## PEARLS AND PITFALLS

- Gel air bubbles can create false pathology, such as a foreign body or vitreous debris
- Frozen gel acts like a gel pad and thus reduces artifact while remaining firm during scan.
- Artifact of hyperechoic lines may appear as a dislocated lens or foreign body when reverberation may be secondary to aquasonic gel. To confirm lens dislocation, observe lens movement with eye motion—artifacts will remain static.

## VIDEOS

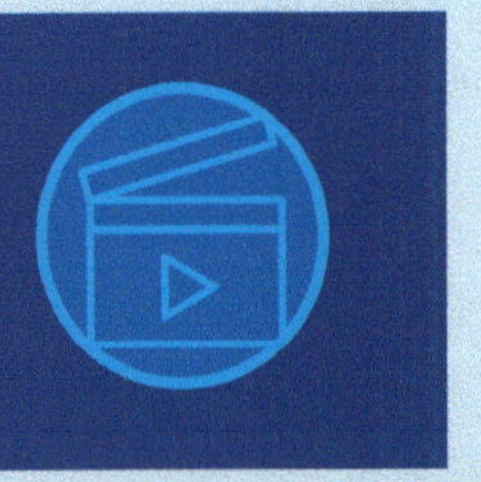

- Ocular Ultrasound

**To access the videos, please go to the List of Videos in the front matter.**

## BIBLIOGRAPHY


Bates, A., & Goett, H. J. (2023). *Ocular ultrasound*. In StatPearls. StatPearls Publishing. https://www.ncbi.nlm.nih.gov/books/NBK459120/

Carroll, D., Elfeky, M., Di Muzio, B., Sharma, R., & McArdle, D. (2024). Posterior vitreous detachment. *Radiopaedia*. Retrieved April 29, 2024, from https://doi.org/10.53347/rID-67864

Chang, M., Finney, N., Baker, J., Rowland, J., Gupta, S., Sarsour, R., Saadat, S., & Fox, J. C. (2023, May 5). Optimal image gain intensity of point-of-care ultrasound when screening for ocular abnormalities in the emergency department. *Western Journal of Emergency Medicine, 24*(3), 622–628. https://doi.org/10.5811/westjem.59714

Di Muzio, B. (2019). Normal eye ultrasound. *Radiopaedia*. Retrieved April 29, 2024, from https://doi.org/10.53347/rID-70415

Gaillard, F., Jones, J., Riahi, P., McArdle, D., & Sharma, R. (2008). Ectopia lentis. *Radiopaedia*. Retrieved April 29, 2024, from https://doi.org/10.53347/rID-1257

Gaillard, F., Di Muzio, B., Elfeky, M., Sharma, R., & McArdle, D. (2008). Retinal detachment. *Radiopaedia*. Retrieved April 29, 2024, from https://doi.org/10.53347/rID-1975

Hacking, C. (2015). Globe rupture. *Radiopaedia*. Retrieved April 29, 2024, from https://doi.org/10.53347/rID-35142

Kerscher, S. R, Tellermann, J., Zipfel, J., Bevot, A., Haas-Lude, K., & Schuhmann, M. U. (2024). Influence of sex and disease etiology on the development of papilledema and optic nerve sheath extension in the setting of intracranial pressure elevation in children. *Brain and Spine, 4*, 102729. https://doi.org/10.1016/j.bas.2023.102729

Soni, N. J., Arntfield, R., & Kory, P. (2020). *Point of care ultrasound* (2nd ed.). Elsevier.

Vaiman, M., Abuita, R., & Bekerman, I. (2015, December 18). Optic nerve sheath diameters in healthy adults measured by computer tomography. *International Journal of Ophthalmology, 8*(6), 1240–1244. https://doi.org/10.3980/j.issn.2222-3959.2015.06.30

# MUSCULOSKELETAL ULTRASOUND

Kelli Craven

## INTRODUCTION

- 90% sensitivity in musculoskeletal (MSK) evaluation
- Highly valuable for tendons, ligaments, cortical fractures, and dislocations
- Tendons comprise 45% of all MSK injuries.
- 66 million MSK injuries occur annually in the US, costing 144 billion dollars.
- Procedural guidance for hematoma and nerve block, arthrocentesis, intra-articular injections
- Identification of osseous erosion, bursitis, tendinopathy, vascularity, dynamic assessment

See Tables 12.1 and 12.2 for indications and differentials.

**Table 12.1** Indications

| Pain | Trauma/injury |
|---|---|
| Redness/swelling/warmth | Deformity |
| Point tenderness | Abnormal physical exam findings |
| Limited range of motion | Procedures |

**Table 12.2** Differentials

| Fracture/dislocation | Chronic disease/injury |
|---|---|
| Septic arthritis | Fluid collection |
| Tendon rupture, tendonitis, tenosynovitis | Bursitis |
| Lipoma versus soft tissue sarcoma (well-defined versus irregular margins) | Gout versus septic arthritis (double contour sign) |

## IMAGE ACQUISITION

- **Probe**
  - Linear probe is ideal for superficial tendons, ligaments, and joints.
  - Curvilinear probe may be necessary for deep structures like the hip or gluteal tendons.

- **Preset**
  - Musculoskeletal

- **Hand placement**
  - "Okay" sign or like a pencil

- **Technique**
  - Image the contralateral side for a comparison of normal versus abnormal.
  - Depending on location of injury, often holding the probe in the "okay" position is most helpful as the small finger and ring finger offer great stability
  - Probe marker toward scanner's left or cephalad in longitudinal view
  - Always image in two planes
  - Measure normal tendon compared to affected tendon
  - To assess tendon or ligament integrity, use:
    - Short-axis view: identifies thickening, tears, or edema
    - Long-axis view: confirms fiber continuity and dynamic motion changes
  - Tendons and ligaments appear as "cars on a highway."
  - In evaluation for fracture or tendon disruption, the probe should be slid up and down, never losing skin contact and always maintaining direct visualization of the cortical and tendon/ligamentous line.

> **PRO TIP**
>
> The probe should be positioned in a true anterior to posterior position. Be mindful that tilting of the probe will create false pathology.

> **PRO TIP**
>
> Do not mistake anisotropy (angle-dependent artifact) for pathology.

- Foreign bodies (e.g., glass, metal, wood) appear hyperechoic with posterior shadowing or reverberation artifact.
  - Wood and organic material: may lack posterior shadowing, requiring high gain settings for detection.

See Table 12.3 for MSK scan protocols.

**Table 12.3** Musculoskeletal Scan Protocols

| MSK Joint | Anatomic Scan Location |
|---|---|
| Shoulder | 1. Bicep tendon. 2. Subscapularis. 3. Infraspinatus. 4. Glenohumeral. 5. Supraspinatus. 6. Acromioclavicular joint |
| Wrist | 1. Doral view (Lister's tubercle and ulna). 2. Longitudinal dorsal view (radius, lunate, capitate, joint capsule). 3. Distal radius view. 4. Ulnar longitudinal. 5. Volar |
| Knee | 1. Suprapatellar. 2. Infrapatellar. 3. Medial. 4. Lateral. 5. Suprapatellar in maximum flexion. 6. Posterior in popliteal crease |
| Ankle | 1. Tibiotalar view. 2. Medial perimalleolar and inframalleolar view. 3. Lateral and inframalleolar view. 4. Achilles tendon at proximal calcaneus view (prone position). 5. Plantar fascia (prone) |

*Source:* Soni, N. J., Arntfield, R., & Kory, P. (2020). *Point of care ultrasound* (2nd ed.). Elsevier.

See Figure 12.1 for MSK anatomy and Figure 12.2 for pathologic MSK anatomy

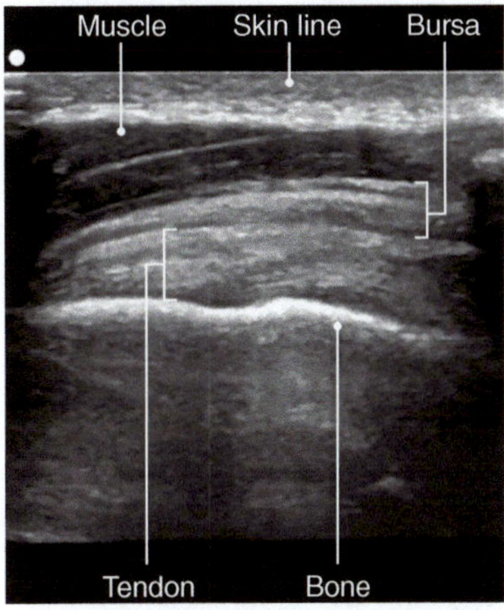


**Figure 12.1.** Normal musculoskeletal anatomy.

*Source:* Image courtesy SonoSim, MSK Core-Clinical, 2024.

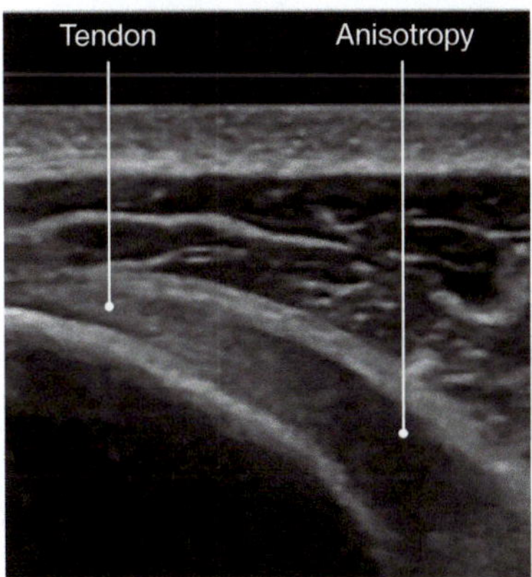


**Figure 12.2.** Anisotropy which is false pathology related to transducer position and imaging angle.

*Source:* Image courtesy SonoSim MSK Closing concepts. summary/closing-concepts, 2024.

## INTERPRETATION

- Most pathology will present with hypoechoic like presentation surrounding a tendon or other soft tissue
- Fractures appear as:
  - Step-off or cortical discontinuity in long bones
  - Echogenic bone fragments in displaced fractures
  - Hematoma formation adjacent to the fracture site
- Osteoarthritis ultrasound findings include:
  - Decreased joint space height
  - Hyperechoic osteophytes
  - Joint effusions or synovial hypertrophy
- Plantar fasciitis findings:
  - Plantar fascia >4 mm thick at calcaneal origin
  - Hypoechoic swelling with loss of normal fibrillar pattern

## PROCEDURE

- **Equipment**
  - Ultrasound machine
  - Gloves
  - Washcloths or towels to wipe up gel
  - Linear probe
- **Patient/scanner position**
  - Patient supine in the position of comfort
  - Joint or area of concern exposed
  - For Achilles tendon scanning
    - Prone with foot hanging off bed (maximal relaxation)
    - Knee slightly flexed to assess dynamic movement
  - For knee ultrasound
    - 30°Flexion: optimal for patellar tendon and joint effusion
    - Full extension: best for meniscal assessment
  - Infraspinatus view: scan posterior to anterior

See Table 12.4 for a summary of pathologic findings.

**Table 12.4** Summary of Pathologic Findings

| Condition | Ultrasound Findings |
|---|---|
| Fracture | Step-off or cortical discontinuity, possible hematoma |
| Tendon rupture | Discontinuity with hypoechoic hematoma, dynamic gapping |
| Bursitis | Anechoic or hypoechoic fluid in bursal space, possible internal debris |
| Arthritis | Decreased joint space height |
| Tendonitis | Diffuse edema, hypoechoic, increased size |
| Osteophyte | Hyperechoic formation, circular in appearance, not part of cortical line, located in a joint space |
| Anisotropy | Hypoechogenic not true pathology |

## PEARLS AND PITFALLS

- Off-axis imaging can create false pathology.

- To avoid anisotropy artifacts: Ensure probe is perpendicular to the tendon fibers

- Reposition probe angle to confirm pathology versus artifact

- Anisotropy of a tendon may lead to misdiagnosis of acute inflammation seen in tendonitis.

- Gentle tension on the Achilles may aid in avoidance of anisotropy.

- Kager's fat pad is naturally hypoechoic. Compare the contralateral side and use color Doppler to differentiate fat pad versus true fluid.

## BIBLIOGRAPHY

Dubey, J., & Shian, B. (2022). Point-of-Care ultrasound for musculoskeletal injection and clinical evaluation. *Primary Care, 49*(1), 163–189. https://doi.org/10.1016/j.pop.2021.10.011

Nakashima, Y., Sunagawa, T., Shinomiya, R., Kodama, A., & Adachi, N. (2022). Point-of-care ultrasound in musculoskeletal field. *Journal of Medical Ultrasonics (2001), 49*(4), 663–673. https://doi.org/10.1007/s10396-022-01252-0

Smallcomb, M., Khandare, S., Vidt, M. E., & Simon, J. C. (2022, August 1). Therapeutic ultrasound and shockwave therapy for tendinopathy: A narrative review. *American Journal of Physical Medicine & Rehabilitation, 101*(8), 801–807. https://doi.org/10.1097/PHM.0000000000001894

# CHAPTER 13

# FIRST TRIMESTER PREGNANCY

Meghan Petzy

## INFORMATION

- Standard of care and expeditious for evaluation in all pregnant patients in the first trimester with abdominal pain and vaginal bleeding in emergency department (ED), clinic, or urgent care setting
- 50% of female patients less likely to receive a diagnostic ultrasound in EDs on nights and weekends
- 99.3% sensitivity for detecting ectopic pregnancy when performed by experienced operators
- Merit-based Incentive Payment System (MIPS) Clinical Quality Measures 2024
  - Ultrasound determination of pregnancy location for pregnant patients with abdominal pain or vaginal bleeding
  - Transabdominal or transvaginal ultrasound for all pregnant patients aged 14 to 50 who present to the ED with a chief complaint of abdominal pain or vaginal bleeding without a documented intrauterine pregnancy (IUP)

See Tables 13.1 and 13.2 for indications and differentials.

**Table 13.1** Indications

| Vaginal bleeding | Pelvic pain | Abdominal pain |
|---|---|---|
| Syncope | Shock | Hemodynamic instability |

**Table 13.2** Differentials

| Early IUP | Ectopic | Subchorionic hemorrhage | Ruptured corpus luteum cyst | Ovarian torsion |
|---|---|---|---|---|
| Intra-abdominal pathologies | Nonviable pregnancy | Infection | Gestational trophoblastic disease | Threatened or spontaneous abortion |

IUP, intrauterine pregnancy.

## IMAGE ACQUISITION

- **Transabdominal technique**
  - Probe
    - Curvilinear
  - Preset
    - Obstetric (OB)
  - Hand placement
    - Hold the probe like a pencil.
  - Probe marker
    - To scanner's left (transverse view), to patient's head (longitudinal view)
  - Patient supine
    - Scanner at patient's side

> **PRO TIP**
>
> Full bladder provides an acoustic window for the uterus and ovaries.

  - Transverse view
    - Bladder in the near field
    - Uterus immediately posterior to the bladder
    - Ovaries on either side of the uterus
    - Tilt superior and inferior to assess uterus from cervix to fundus
  - Longitudinal view
    - Pubic bone top right of the screen
    - Bladder posterior to the pubic bone
    - Uterus posterior to the bladder with endometrial stripe, uterine fundus, cervix, vaginal strip
    - Fan left to right to obtain cross-sectional views of the uterus
    - Slide probe to either side and aim laterally to visualize ovaries (lie adjacent and medial to external iliac vessels)

## IMAGE ACQUISITION

- **Transvaginal technique**
  - Probe
    - Endocavitary
  - Preset
    - OB
  - Hand placement
    - Thumb on top and fingers underneath

- Probe marker
  - Toward the ceiling (longitudinal view), rotate 90° Counterclockwise (coronal view)
- Patient supine
  - Scanner at foot of bed or at side of patient

---

**PRO TIP**

Scan on an empty bladder when in transvaginal mode.

---

- Gel is applied to the transducer, then a sterile probe cover, then sterile gel
- Insert into vaginal canal
- Longitudinal view
  - Bladder in the near field on the left of the screen
  - Endometrial stripe seen toward the cervix
  - Fan side to side to view the entire uterus
  - Cervix and pouch of Douglas are seen by aiming posteriorly from the midline (assessing for free fluid)
  - Tilt laterally toward pelvic walls to assess ovaries (iliac vessels adjacent to ovaries)
- Coronal view
  - Return to the midline, rotate counterclockwise 90°
  - Only the uterus may be visible
  - Direct beam laterally and obliquely to locate ovaries

## ANATOMY/IMAGES

See Figures 13.1 through 13.5

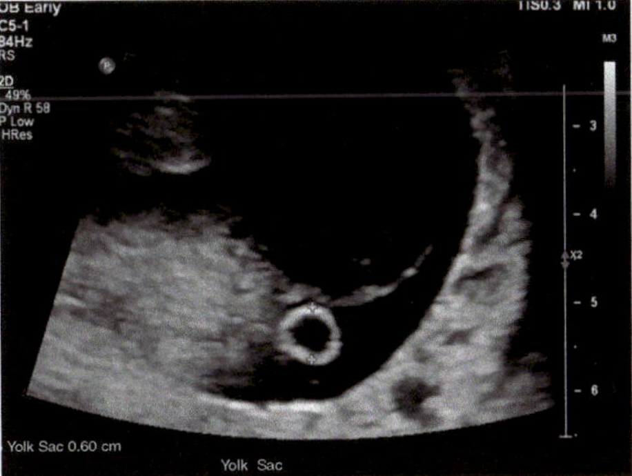


**Figure 13.1.** Confirmed intrauterine pregnancy with yolk sac.

*Source:* Used with permission. Image courtesy of M. Petzy.

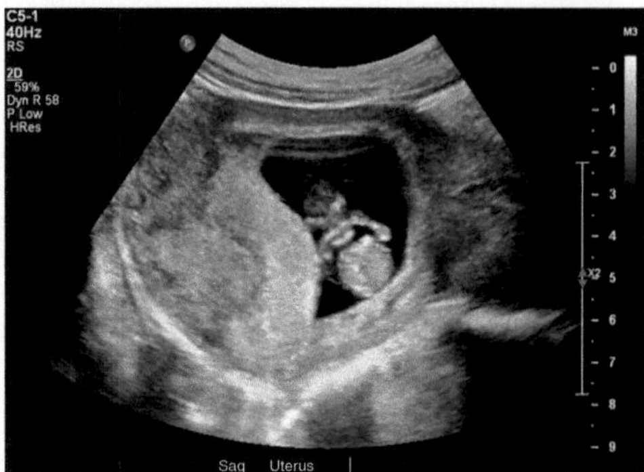

**Figure 13.2.** Confirmed transabdominal intrauterine pregnancy in first trimester.

*Source:* Used with permission. Image courtesy of M. Petzy.

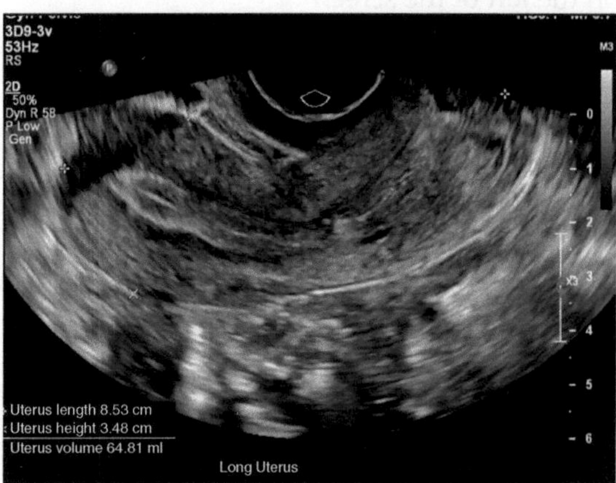

**Figure 13.3.** Intracavitary probe: longitudinal uterus.

*Source:* Used with permission. Image courtesy of M. Petzy.

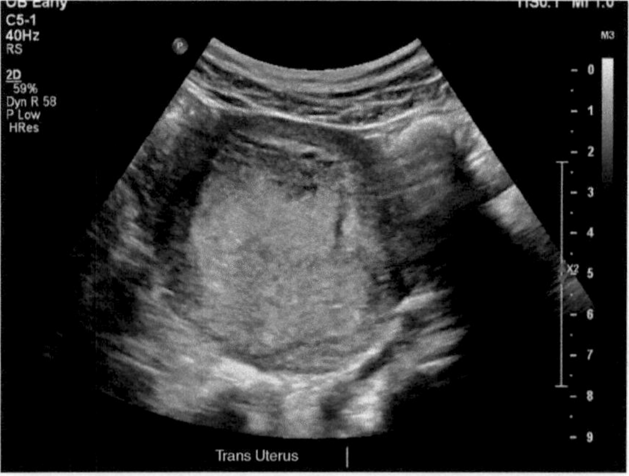

**Figure 13.4.** Transabdominal transverse uterus.

*Source:* Used with permission. Image courtesy of M. Petzy.

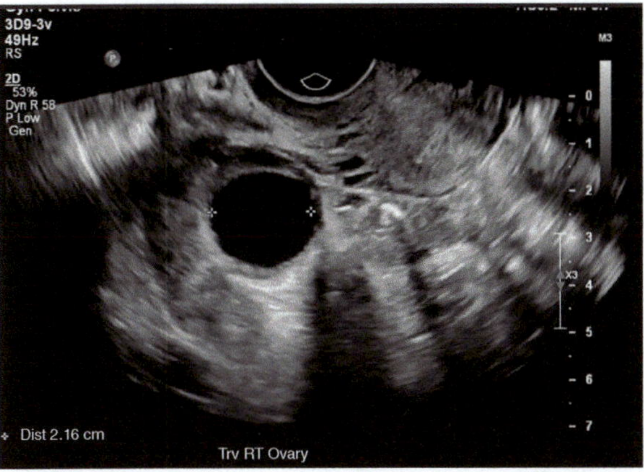


**Figure 13.5.** Transvaginal right ovarian cyst with intracavitary probe.

*Source:* Used with permission. Image courtesy of M. Petzy.

## INTERPRETATION

Ultrasound landmarks by gestational age

- 4.5 to 5 weeks: gestational sac visible (round, anechoic, with hyperechoic ring)
- 5 to 6 weeks: yolk sac appears within the gestational sac
- 6 to 7 weeks: fetal pole with cardiac activity

Definitive IUP requires:

- Gestational sac located in the fundus or mid-uterus
- Yolk sac present (confirms early pregnancy)
- Fetal pole with cardiac activity (>100 bpm at 6 weeks, 110–175 bpm later)

See Table 13.3 for a summary of first trimester pregnancy pathologic findings.

**Table 13.3** First Trimester Pregnancy Summary of Pathologic Findings

| Condition | Ultrasound Findings |
| --- | --- |
| IUP | Yolk sac in an intrauterine gestational sac; fetal heart rate (110–175 bpm); crown-rump length; located at the uterine fundus, elliptical shape, eccentric to the endometrium, decidual reaction (FEEDS)<br>Round, thin-walled echogenic ring with anechoic center = yolk sac<br>Anechoic, circular, or oval structure with surrounding echogenic ring = gestational sac<br>Round mass adjacent to yolk sac seen after 5 weeks = fetal pole or embryo<br>Amniotic sac without embryo = failed pregnancy |
| Amion or blighted ovum | Anechoic space within the gestational sac seen by 7 weeks<br>Gestational sac >25 mm with no yolk sac or fetal pole.<br>Absent cardiac activity at >7 mm CRL |
| Intrauterine device (IUD) | T-shaped hyperechoic echogenic structure in the uterus<br>**Pro Tip**: IUD + pregnancy test = high suspicion for ectopic pregnancy |
| Corpus luteum cyst | Hypoechoic area within the ovary, free fluid pelvis/abdomen, NEGATIVE HCG |
| Subchorionic hemorrhage | Fluid collection between chorionic margin and uterine wall (anechoic or echogenic) crescent-like appearance |
| Gestational trophoblastic disease | Complex, cystic, hypervascular intrauterine mass = "cluster of grapes" |

*(continued)*

**Table 13.3** First Trimester Pregnancy Summary of Pathologic Findings (*continued*)

| Heterotopic pregnancy | IUP + ectopic pregnancy<br>History of fertility treatment |
|---|---|
| Ectopic pregnancy | No IUP, HCG positive HCG, beta-HCG >1,500 mIU/mL, tubal ring sign (echogenic ring with hypoechoic center), irregular adnexal mass<br>Visualized gestational sac with yolk sac or embryo outside the uterus |
| Ruptured ectopic pregnancy | Moderate to large free fluid in pelvis/abdomen, pregnant with acute abdomen, diffuse abdominal pain, syncope, hemodynamic instability<br>Obtain a FAST exam |

CRL, crown-rump length; IUP, intrauterine pregnancy.

## PEARLS AND PITFALLS

- Transabdominal and transvaginal views recommended
  - If the transabdominal scan shows IUP, transvaginal views may not be needed
- Identification of gestational sac is detected earlier with a transvaginal scan
- Transabdominal = full bladder; transvaginal = empty bladder
- Ovaries can be difficult to see on transabdominal views due to bowel gas, use slight compression of bowel to displace
- Pregnant patient
  - A small amount of physiologic free fluid is expected in the cul-de-sac.
  - Do not overlook other etiologies (ruptured cyst, ovarian torsion).
- Rule in an IUP versus rule out an ectopic and obtain beta-HCG
- Pregnant patient + hemoperitoneum + no IUP = ruptured ectopic pregnancy
- When in doubt, seek diagnostic ultrasound and OB/GYN consultation

## VIDEOS

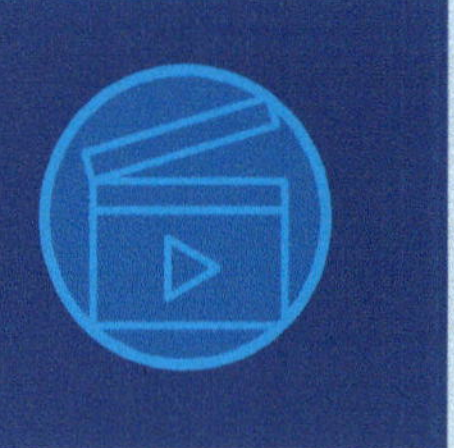

- Transabdominal View
- First Trimester Pregnancy

**To access the videos, please go to the List of Videos in the front matter.**

## BIBLIOGRAPHY

Centers for Medicare & Medicaid Services. (2023, December). *Quality ID #254: Ultrasound determination of pregnancy location for pregnant patients with abdominal pain or vaginal bleeding.* Quality Measures: Traditional MIPS Requirements. https://qpp.cms.gov/docs/QPP_quality_measure_specifications/CQM-Measures/2023_Measure_254_MIPSCQM.pdf

Soni, N. J., Arntfield, R., & Kory, P. (2020). *Point of care ultrasound* (2nd ed.). Elsevier.

# CHAPTER 14

# PEDIATRIC ULTRASOUND

Kelli Craven

## INTRODUCTION

- Intussusception affects 50 per 100,000 children annually. The classic triad (intermittent abdominal pain, bloody stools, and a palpable "sausage-shaped" mass) is present in <50% of cases.
- Ultrasound is the first-line imaging modality and gold standard for diagnosing intussusception (Zabadayev, 2022).
- Appendicitis common between 10 and 30 years of age with US sensitivity/specificity comparable to CT.
- Procedural guidance with US is becoming standard of care and demonstrates similar efficacy
- Pediatric specific scans: lung, abdominal, cranial, spinal, cardiac

See Tables 14.1 and 14.2 for indications and differentials.

**Table 14.1** Indications

| Bilious emesis/vomiting | Abdominal pain/masses |
| --- | --- |
| Abnormal physical exam | Bloody stools |
| Trauma/injury | Eye pain |
| Airway compromise | Procedures [LP, IV access, intubation] |

LP, lumbar puncture.

**Table 14.2** Differentials

| Intussusception | Pyloric stenosis |
| --- | --- |
| Appendicitis | Ophthalmic injuries |
| Infectious | Cardiac anomalies |
| E-FAST/pneumothorax | Intracranial hemorrhage |

## IMAGE ACQUISITION

- **Probe**
  - Curvilinear: best for deep abdominal structures (e.g., intussusception, pyloric stenosis)
  - Linear: preferred for superficial structures (e.g., appendix, soft tissue, vascular access)
  - Phased array: used for cardiac and lung assessments.
- **Preset**
  - Abdominal for pyloric stenosis, appendix, and intussusception evaluation
- **Hand placement**
  - "Okay" sign or hold like a pencil
- **Technique**
  - Always maintain the proper position of the probe marker to determine proper planes and anatomical position
  - Cardiac assessment using the phased array probe and selecting the cardiac exam type places the screen marker dot on the right; if not in cardiac mode the screen marker dot is on the left.
  - Ophthalmic views obtained same as an adult exam
  - E-FAST exam in pediatrics is same as adult
  - Cardiac views obtained same as adult exam
  - Lumbar puncture, peripheral IV, and intubation views obtained same as adult exam
  - Intussusception
    - View the entire ascending, transverse, and descending colon for intussusception

> **PRO TIP**
>
> Start in the right lower quadrant (RLQ) and scan cephalad.

    - Transverse and longitudinal views with measurements must be acquired for all exams and suspicious appearing bowel wall findings.
  - Appendix
    - Views are best obtained starting the scan in mid right abdomen, gently compressing in a gradient fashion moving bowel and bowel gas out of view, sliding the probe down toward RLQ where the tubular structure is noted to overlie the psoas muscle and iliac vessel
    - Should appear as a blind-ended pouch
    - Appendicoliths will have a hyperechoic finding with shadowing much like a renal or gallbladder stone.

> **PRO TIP**
>
> The clinician may also have the patient point to the area of maximal tenderness for a scanning point.

- Pyloric stenosis
  - Best found in right upper quadrant (RUQ) where antrum of the stomach meets the pylorus using the liver as a viewing window

## ANATOMY/IMAGES

See Figures 14.1 through 14.4 for images of appendicitis findings, intussusception, and pyloric stenosis.

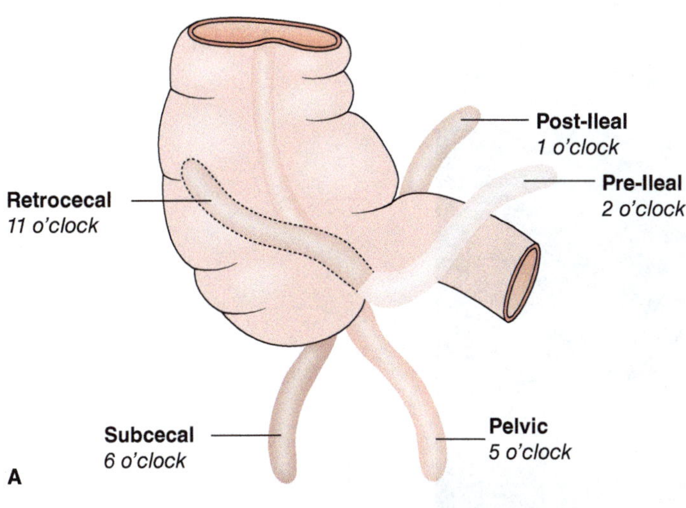


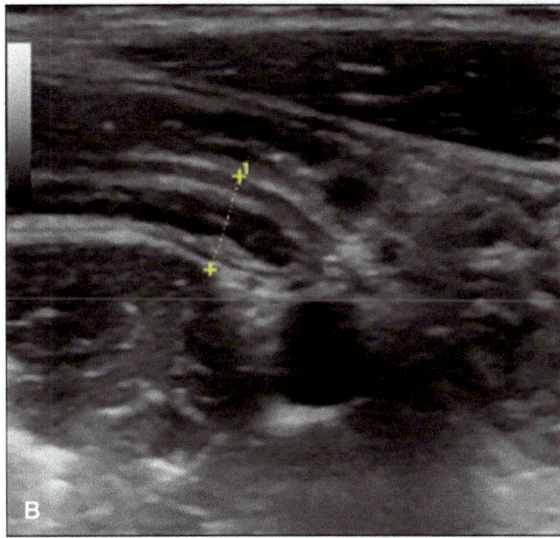


**Figure 14.1.** Normal appendix presentation and anatomical locations. (A) Anatomical positions of appendix. (B) Normal appendix longitudinal view.

*Source:* Tooma, D., Dinh, V., Ahn, J., Deschamps, J., Genobaga, S., Lang, A., Lee, V., Krause, R., & White, S. (n.d.). *Abdominal ultrasound made easy: Step-by-step guide.* POCUS 101. https://www.pocus101.com /abdominal-ultrasound-made-easy-step-by-step-guide/#Pediatric_Abdominal_Ultrasound_Applications. Images used with permission.

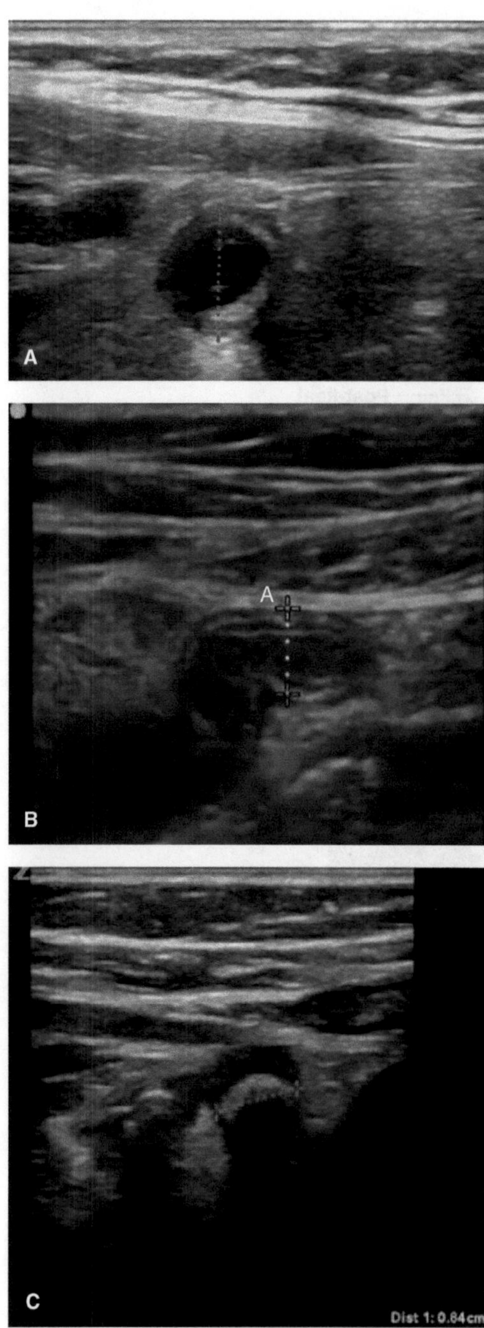

**Figure 14.2.** Appendicitis findings. (A) "Target" sign. (B) Dilated appendix with blind ended pouch. (C) Appendicoliths appear hyperechoic and will cast a shadow within the lumen.

*Source:* Tooma, D., Dinh, V., Ahn, J., Deschamps, J., Genobaga, S., Lang, A., Lee, V., Krause, R., & White, S. (n.d.). *Abdominal ultrasound made easy: Step-by-step guide.* POCUS 101. https://www.pocus101.com /abdominal-ultrasound-made-easy-step-by-step-guide/#Pediatric_Abdominal_Ultrasound_Applications. Images used with permission.

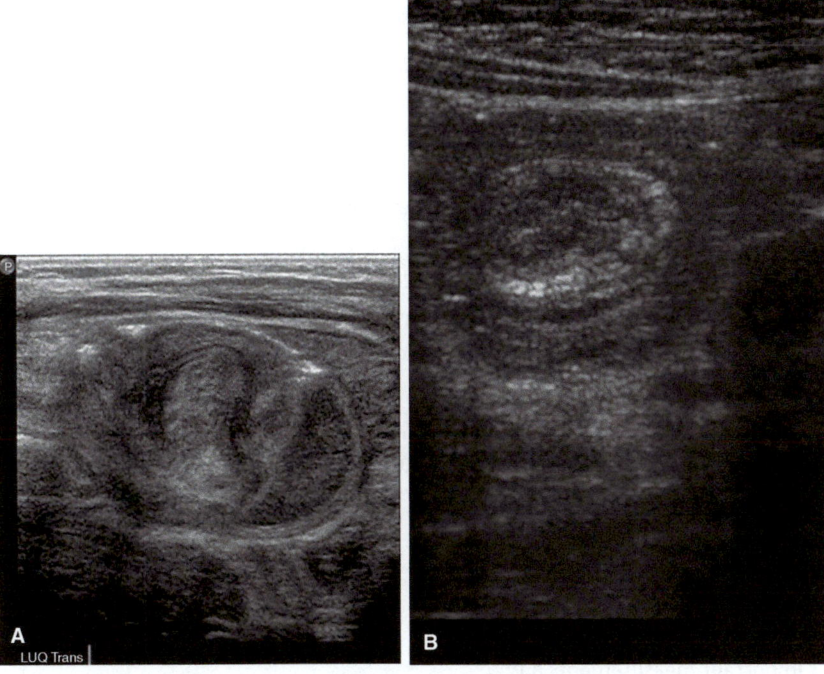

**Figure 14.3.** Intussusception. (A). Pseudokidney sign. (B) Donut sign.

*Source:* Tooma, D., Dinh, V., Ahn, J., Deschamps, J., Genobaga, S., Lang, A., Lee, V., Krause, R., & White, S. (n.d.). *Abdominal ultrasound made easy: Step-by-step guide.* POCUS 101. https://www.pocus101.com/abdominal -ultrasound-made-easy-step-by-step-guide/#Pediatric_Abdominal_Ultrasound_Applications. Images used with permission

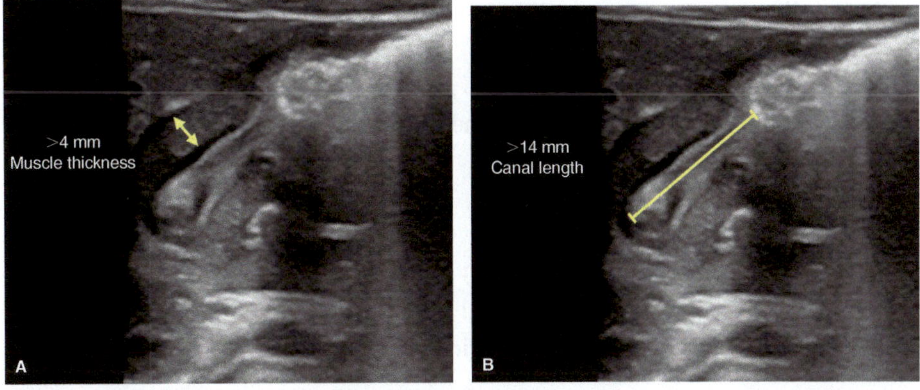


**Figure 14.4.** Pyloric stenosis findings. (A) Pyloric muscularis diameter. (B) Pyloric canal Length.

*Source:* Tooma, D., Dinh, V., Ahn, J., Deschamps, J., Genobaga, S., Lang, A., Lee, V., Krause, R., & White, S. (n.d.). *Abdominal ultrasound made easy: Step-by-step guide.* POCUS 101. https://www.pocus101.com /abdominal-ultrasound-made-easy-step-by-step-guide/#Pediatric_Abdominal_Ultrasound_Applications. Images used with permission

## INTERPRETATION

### Interpretation

- Intussusception presents like a "target" sign.
  - Ileocecal intussusception
    - Location RLQ
    - Will measure >2 cm × 3 cm
    - Absent normal appearing ileocecal junction
    - Thickened cecal wall
    - Increased blood flow on color Doppler
    - Decreased blood flow and surrounding edema within the intussusception
      - Surgical consult versus interventional radiology (IR)
      - May represent necrosis
    - Lymph node like appearance in longitudinal view
    - Hyperechoic findings inside the target represent mesenteric fat
- Pyloric stenosis demonstrates "doughnut" sign
  - Diagnostic measurements
    - Muscularis externa >3 mm

---

**PRO TIP**

The most important measurements are:

- Pyloric transverse >14 mm.
- Pyloric lumen length >15 to 17 mm.

---

**PRO TIP**

Remember that Pi = 3.1416 equals muscularis externa > 3mm and pyloric canal > 14–16mm.

---

- **Appendix**
  - Location RLQ
  - Thickened wall
  - Edema/ hypoechoic findings in the lumen
  - Fat stranding
  - Measurement
    - <6 mm normal diameter
    - >8 mm abnormal diameter
    - >3 mm wall thickness abnormal

See Table 14.3 for summary of pathologic findings.

**Table 14.3** Summary of Pathologic Findings

| Condition | Ultrasound Findings |
|---|---|
| Intussusception | "Target" sign, increased cecum wall<br>Longitudinal image represents a "lymph node" like appearance, may have increased or decreased blood flow on color Doppler, might have evidence of free fluid, RLQ or LLQ, lymph nodes may be pulled into the intussusception |
| Pyloric stenosis | "Donut" sign, measurement of muscularis externa > 3mm and canal length > 14mm |
| Free fluid | Hypoechoic presentation as seen in ascites and may be seen in various quadrants |
| Appendicitis | Fat stranding, increased diameter > 6mm, edema, thickened wall > 3mm, stone with shadow |

RLQ, right lower quadrant; LLQ, left lower quadrant.

## PEARLS AND PITFALLS

- Ileocecal intussusception must be reduced to prevent bowel ischemia and subsequent perforation of bowel wall.
- Use caudal tip of the liver for increased viewing of pylorus
- May need to put child in the right lateral decubitus position to remove bowel gas
- Wait 15 minutes if child has ingested milk to decrease chance of gas pathology prior to evaluating pylorus.

## BIBLIOGRAPHY

Costa, D. S., Swinson, S., Torrão, H., Gonçalves, L., Kurochka, S., Pina Vaz, C., & Mendes, V. (2012). Hypertrophic pyloric stenosis: Tips and tricks for ultrasound diagnosis. *Insights Imaging, 3*, 247–250. https://doi.org/10.1007/s13244-012-0168-x

Farrow, R. (2024). *5 minute sono: Pyloric stenosis* [Video]. YouTube. Retrieved July 10, 2024, from https://www.youtube.com/watch?app=desktop&v=_hvzmgbTDxI

Lin-Martore, M., Kornblith, A. E., Kohn, M. A., & Gottlieb, M. (2020). Diagnostic accuracy of point-of-care ultrasound for intussusception in children presenting to the emergency department: A systematic review and meta-analysis. *Western Journal of Emergency Medicine, 21*(4), 1008–1016. https://doi.org/10.5811/westjem.2020.4.46241

Owen, J. W. (2021). *Ultrasound for suspected appendicitis in children*. Retrieved July 10, 2024, from https://www.youtube.com/watch?v=VO51vgSEXuE

Yehouenou, T. R. T., El, H. S., Oze, K. R., Mohamed Traore, W. Y., Dinga Ekadza, J. A., Allali, N., & Chat, L. (2021). A child's acute intestinal intussusception and literature review. *Global Pediatric Health, 8*. https://doi.org/10.1177/2333794X211059110

Zabadayev, S. (2022). *Pediatric abdominal ultrasound: Part 1*. [Image 13.1 B, C]. [Video]. *POCUS 101*. YouTube. Retrieved December 26, 2024, from https://www.youtube.com/watch?v=uVjkCS95wl4&t=50s

# CHAPTER 15

# SHOCK—RAPID ULTRASOUND FOR SHOCK AND HYPOTENSION PROTOCOL

John Barrett

## INTRODUCTION

- Rapid ultrasound for shock and yypotension (RUSH) is the most commonly used protocol for rapid assessment of undifferentiated hypotension.
- In undifferentiated shock, RUSH improved diagnostic accuracy from 60.6% to 85% and changed management in 50% of patients (Ramadan et al., 2023).
- HI-MAP mnemonic (heart, inferior vena cava [IVC], Morison's pouch, aorta, pulmonary) is helpful for remembering the RUSH protocol.

See Table 15.1 for indications and Table 15.2 for differentials.

**Table 15.1** Indications

| Hemodynamic instability | Tachycardia/bradycardia | Abdominal pain |
|---|---|---|
| Trauma/injury | Respiratory distress/failure | Fever |

**Table 15.2** Categories of Shock

| Type | Cause |
|---|---|
| **Distributive** | Septic<br>Neurogenic<br>Anaphylactic |
| **Hypovolemic** | Trauma<br>Gastrointestinal bleeding<br>Postpartum<br>Diarrhea<br>Burns |
| **Cardiogenic** | Myocardial infarction<br>Cardiomyopathy<br>Heart failure<br>Arrythmias<br>Structural heart disease |
| **Obstructive** | Pulmonary embolism<br>Pericardial tamponade<br>Tension pneumothorax |

## PROTOCOL

See Table 15.3 for a description of the protocol.

**Table 15.3** Protocol

| Pneumonic | Organ/System | POCUS Evaluation |
|---|---|---|
| H | Heart | Ejection fraction<br>Right ventricle strain with pulmonary embolism<br>Pericardial effusion and tamponade |
| I | IVC | Size<br>Collapsibility |
| M | Morison's Pouch | Peritoneal free fluid |
| A | Aorta | Abdominal aortic aneurysm |
| P | Pulmonary | Pneumothorax |

IVC, inferior vena cava; POCUS, point-of-care ultrasound.

## TRANSDUCER

- **Phased array**

## HEART

- **Views**
  - Parasternal long axis (PLAX)
  - Parasternal short axis (PSSA)
  - Apical 4 chamber (A4C)
  - Subxiphoid/subcostal
- **Assessment**
  - Assessing for left ventricular (LV) systolic function (visual estimation, E-point septal separation)
  - Detecting pericardial effusion (fluid collection, tamponade physiology)
  - Evaluating right ventricular (RV) strain
- **Pathology**
  - Pericardial effusion
    - Detection of anechoic/hypoechoic fluid around the heart
    - Right atrial and RV collapse during diastole suggestive of tamponade
  - Right heart strain
    - RV enlargement, septal flattening, and D-shaped LV ("D" sign)
    - Assess for McConnell's sign (apical sparing with RV hypokinesis) in pulmonary embolism.
  - Left ventricular function
    - Estimation of ejection fraction based on ventricular wall motion
    - Hyperdynamic LV in early hypovolemic or septic shock, before decompensation

## ■ Examples

- Figure 15.1. Pulmonary hypertension

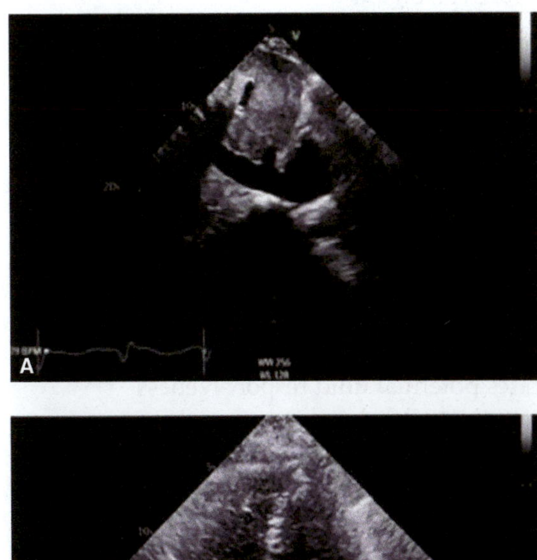

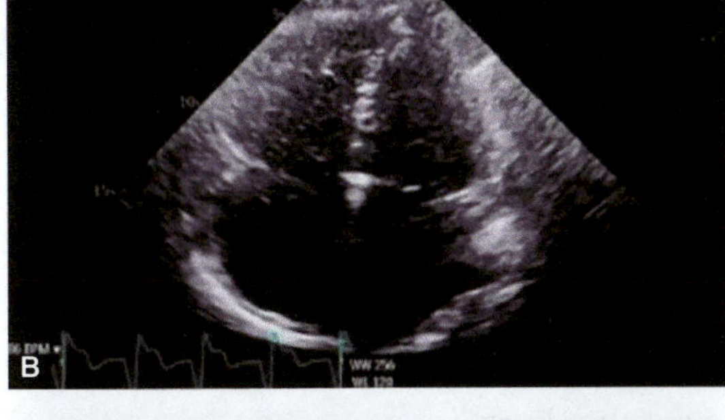

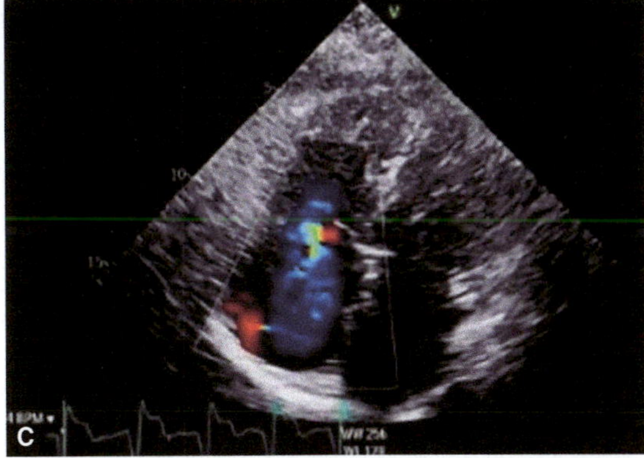

**Figure 15.1.** Images representative of pulmonary hypertension. (**A**) Dilated inferior vena cava. (**B**) Enlarged right atrium. Note cardiac preset. (**C**) Severe tricuspid regurgitation. Note cardiac preset.

*Source:* Yu Jia Ke, D., Tso, M., Johri, A. M. (2024). The application of point of care ultrasound to screen for pulmonary hypertension: A narrative review. *POCUS Journal, 9*(1): 109–116. Retrieved from https://pocusjournal.com/article/17494/

## INFERIOR VENA CAVA

- **Views**
  - Subxiphoid longitudinal and transverse view
- **Assessment**
  - Measuring IVC diameter and assessing collapsibility with respiration
  - IVC collapsibility of >50% suggests fluid responsiveness in spontaneously breathing patients, but interpretation differs in ventilated patients.
- **Interpretation**
  - IVC diameter and collapsibility suggest volume status
    - IVC <2.1 cm + >50% collapse → fluid responsive
    - IVC >2.1 cm + <50% collapse → elevated central venous pressure, possible fluid overload
  - A small, collapsible IVC indicates potential fluid responsiveness.
  - A large, noncollapsible IVC suggests high central venous pressure and possible fluid overload.

## MORISON'S POUCH AND FAST EXAM VIEWS

- **Views**
  - Right upper quadrant (RUQ)
  - Left upper quadrant (LUQ)
  - Pelvis
  - Thoracic windows for pleural effusions
- **Assessment**
  - Free fluid in trauma patients suggests hemoperitoneum, while in nontraumatic cases, it may indicate ascites, ruptured ectopic pregnancy, or peritoneal dialysis leak. Identify free fluid in the abdomen and thoracic cavities which may indicate hemorrhage or pleural effusion.
- **Pathology**
  - Detection of anechoic fluid collections in the abdomen (hemoperitoneum) or thorax (hemothorax/pleural effusion)
  - Look for the spine sign (thoracic spine visible above the diaphragm) to confirm pleural effusion or hemothorax.
- **Examples**
  - Figure 15.2. Right upper quadrant

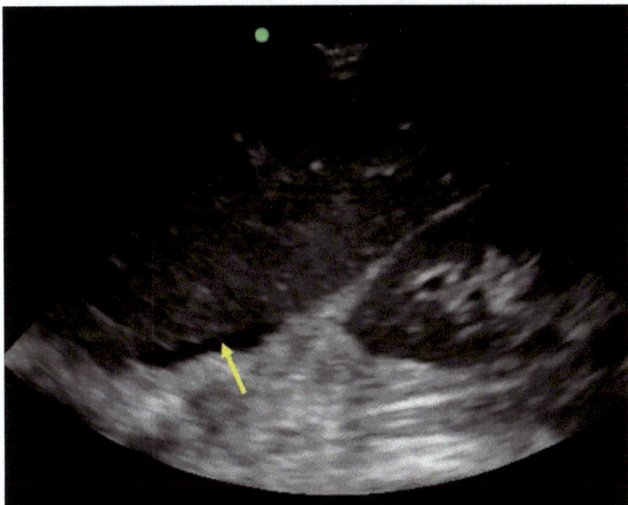

**Figure 15.2.** Right upper quadrant demonstrates anechoic fluid near the liver border (yellow arrow).

*Source:* Douglas, S., Newbigging, J., & Robertson, D. (2016). Case report: FAST ultrasound interpretation in trauma resuscitation. *POCUS Journal 1*(3), 13–14. Retrieved from https://pocusjournal.com/article/2016-01-03p13-14/

## AORTA AND ANEURYSM

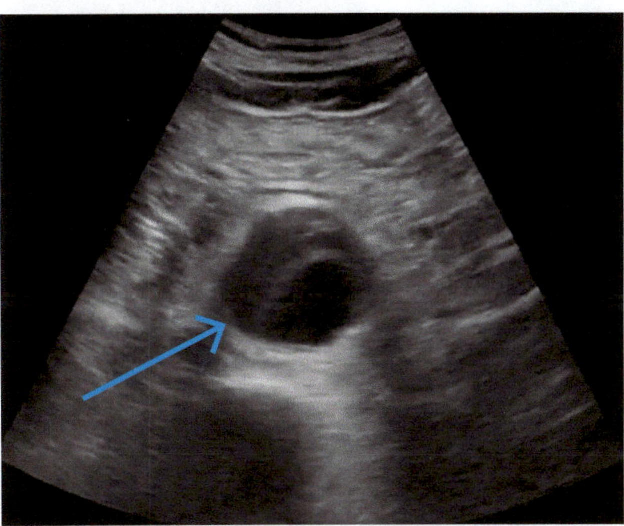

**Figure 15.3.** Infrarenal 5.0 x 5.3 cm abdominal aortic aneurysm (denoted by blue arrow). True lumen hypoechoic.

*Source:* Seu, R., Gartenberg, A., Mirsky, R., Bandagi, A., Leonard-Shiu, N. J., Panjwani, R., McNulty, N., Dixon, T., Montenegro, M. A., & Halperin, M. (2025). Point of care ultrasound (POCUS) used to rapidly diagnose both renal colic and a symptomatic abdominal aortic aneurysm in an elderly man with left flank pain. *POCUS Journal, 10*(1), 131–133. Retrieved from https://pocusjournal.com/article/18461/

- **Views**
  - Transverse and longitudinal views of the abdominal aorta
- **Assessment**
  - Suspected aortic aneurysm or dissection (cannot rule out dissection)
- **Pathology**
  - Normal aortic diameter: <3.0 cm
  - Aneurysm: >3.0 cm
  - High rupture risk: >5.5 cm (requires surgical intervention), aneurysm detection with an aortic diameter >3 cm.

**PRO TIP**

Point-of-care ultrasound (POCUS) cannot rule out aortic dissection, but look for:

- Intimal flap (mobile echogenic line in lumen).
- Aortic dilation with asymmetric flow on Doppler.

- Signs of aortic rupture or dissection, such as retroperitoneal hematoma or intraluminal flap
- **Examples**
  - Figure 15.3. Aneurysm
  - Figure 15.4. Pelvis

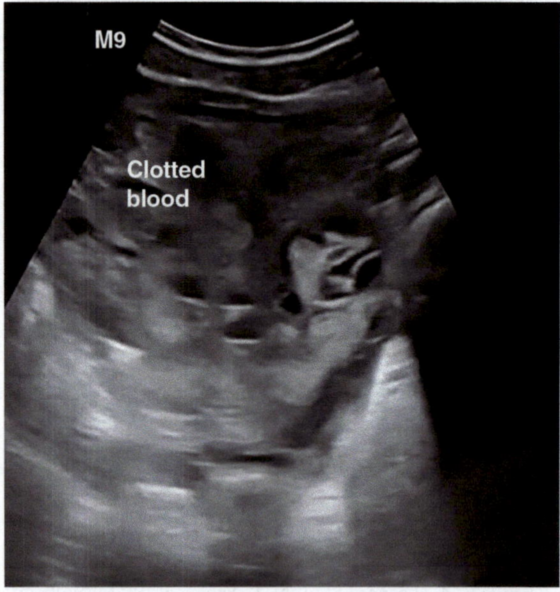


**Figure 15.4.** Clotted blood noted in transverse view of pelvis.

*Source:* Lammers, S., Hong, C, Tepper, J., Moore, C., Baston, C., & Dolin, C. D. (2021). Use of point-of-care ultrasound to diagnose spontaneous rupture of fibroid in pregnancy. *POCUS Journal, 6*(1):16–21. https://doi.org/10.24908/pocus.v6i1.14757

## PULMONARY

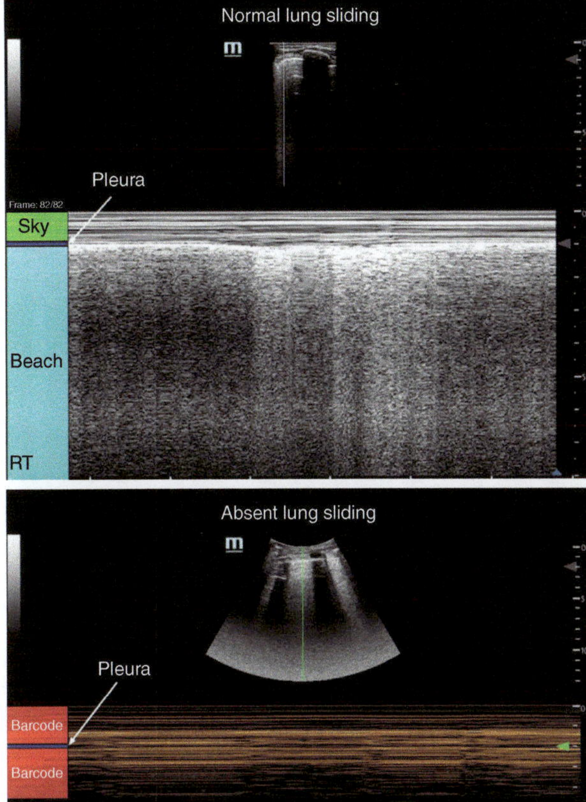


**Figure 15.5.** Pneumothorax.

*Source:* Used with permission from the University of Pennsylvania Health System, Ultrasound Division.

- **Views**
  - Anterior chest for pneumothorax
  - Lateral chest for pleural effusion
- **Assessment**
  - Suspected pneumothorax
- **Image acquisition**
  - Techniques
    - Lung sliding and B-lines assessment using a high-frequency linear transducer
    - Consider M-mode (seashore versus barcode sign) for pneumothorax confirmation

- ■ **Pathology**
  - Absence of lung sliding and the presence of a "barcode sign" or "stratosphere sign" seen in pneumothorax
  - Absence of lung sliding could also be lack of breathing, main stem intubation, or patient with pleurodesis

See Figure 15.5 for images on normal and absent lung siding.

## PEARLS AND PITFALLS

- ■ IVC dilation in ventilated patients may not always indicate volume overload—correlate with clinical exam and cardiac function.
- ■ Differentiate by checking if fluid is anterior to the descending aorta (pericardial) versus posterior (pleural effusion).
- ■ If subxiphoid view is difficult, use PLAX or A4C as alternatives.

## BIBLIOGRAPHY

Ramadan, A., Abdallah, T., Abdelsalam, H., Mokhtar, A., & Razek, A. A. (2023). Evaluation of parameters used in echocardiography and ultrasound protocol for the diagnosis of shock etiology in emergency setting. *BMC Emergency Medicine, 23*, 132. https://doi.org/10.1186/s12873-023-00902-x

# CHAPTER 16

# VASCULAR ACCESS

Adriana De La Rue

## INTRODUCTION

- Ultrasound-guided IV access results in reliable medication access and source for recurrent blood draws, improving patient satisfaction.
- Ultrasound-guided central venous catheter (CVC) placement can improve first attempt success by 57% (Genobaga et al., n.d.) while limiting complications by 71% (Genobaga et al., n.d.) (e.g., arterial puncture, bleeding, hematoma).
- Central venous catheter lines are nontunnelled percutaneous catheters placed in either the left or right internal jugular, subclavian, or common femoral veins.
- Peripheral intravenous catheter placement is a tool that can be utilized in patients with poor vasculature and venous access.

See Table 16.1 for indications for US-guided peripheral and central venous access.

**Table 16.1** Indications for US Guided Peripheral and Central Venous Access

| | |
|---|---|
| Limited IV access | Multiple failed IV attempts |
| Vascular diseases | Comorbidities: ESRD, DM, sickle Cell, IVDU |
| Hemodynamic monitoring | Mass transfusion of multiple blood products |
| Infusion of certain medications ie., vasopressors | Emergent dialysis catheter placement |
| ECMO | Transvenous pacing |

DM, diabetes mellitus; ECMO, extracorporeal membrane oxygenation; ESRD, end-stage renal disease; IVDU, IV drug use.

## IMAGE ACQUISITION

- **Probe**
  - Linear probe for all vascular access (high-frequency and high-resolution)
  - Vascular preset
- **Hand placement**
  - Use dominant hand during initial identification and selection of vein
  - Transition probe to nondominant hand and hold like a pencil
  - Stabilize the probe with the middle, ring, and small fingers
  - Use dominant hand for all vascular access

## ■ Technique

- Basic principles of vascular selection
  - ○ Artery: less compressible, more pulsatile
  - ○ Vein: more compressible, less pulsatile
  - ○ Apply color flow and/or pulse wave Doppler to distinguish between artery and vein
- Other considerations
  - ○ Evaluate skin for overlying cellulitis, history of thrombosis, prior CVC cannulation, or vessel trauma.
- CVC sites
  - ○ Internal jugular (IJ) vein: the right IJ is preferred over the left IJ secondary to larger diameter and more lateral of the common carotid

### PRO TIP

Internal jugular vein is lateral to the common carotid artery.

  - ○ Subclavian vein has lower risk of infection
  - ○ Femoral vein and artery
    - – Femoral vein is within femoral triangle, medial to the femoral artery and nerve and inferior to the inguinal ligament
    - – Recommended puncture site is proximal to saphenous vein but inferior to inguinal ligament

## ANATOMY/IMAGES

Figure 16.1 illustrates the proper and improper methods to access vessel with a needle tip. See Figure 16.2 for information on imaging of a CVC. Figure 16.3 provides information on needle tip visualization.

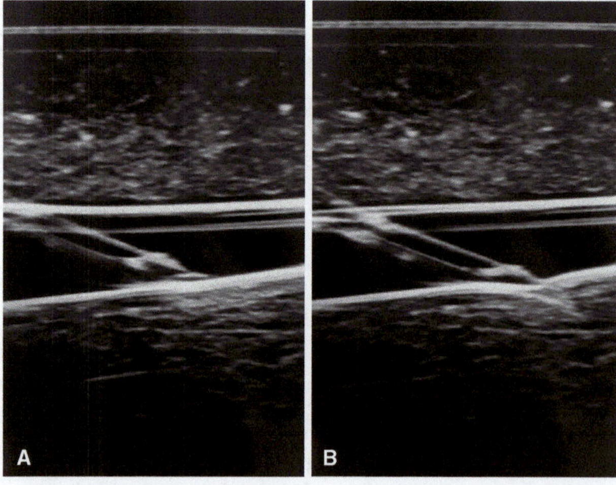


**Figure 16.1.** Vessel access. (A) Proper access with needle tip inside vessel. (B) Improper access as needle tip is through vessel wall.

*Source*: Used with permission from Adriana De La Rue, PA-C.

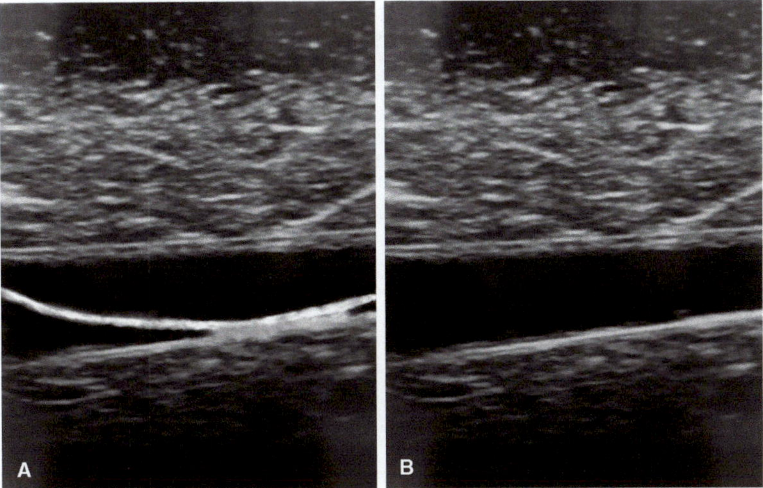

**Figure 16.2.** Central venous catheter. (A) Guidewire inside vessel. (B) No evidence of guidewire.
*Source*: Used with permission from Adriana De La Rue, PA-C.

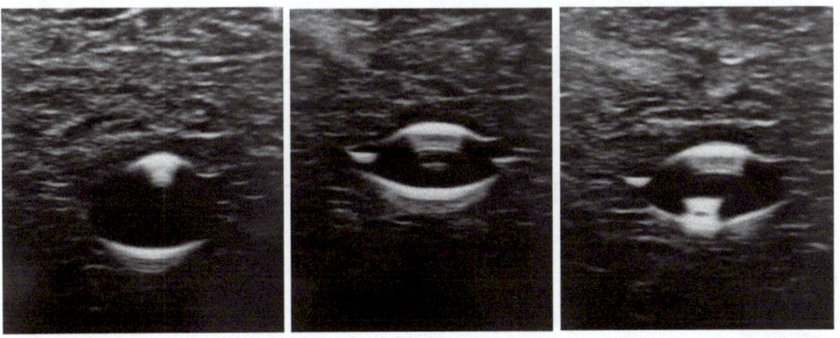

**Figure 16.3.** Needle tip visualization. (A) Hyperchoic needle tip visualized within vein lumen. (B) Catheter visualized within the vein lumen, resting on the inferior aspect.
*Source*: Images used with permission from Adriana De La Rue, PA-C.

## INTERPRETATION

- Visualize hyperechoic line (catheter) or needle tip within vein in both the transverse and longitudinal views.
- Following peripheral IV cannulation, the catheter should be visualized resting on the inferior aspect of the vein.
- If color flow is added, artery will be pulsatile even if compressible

## PROCEDURE

- **Equipment**
  - CVC
    - Linear probe

- ○ Sterile probe covers
- ○ Central line kit
  - – Sterile gown and gloves
  - – Chloraprep
  - – Sterile drapes
  - – Sterile saline flushes
  - – 25G injection needle
  - – Lidocaine 1%
  - – 18G Introducer needle
  - – 10 mL syringe
  - – J-tip Guide Wire
  - – Triple lumen catheter
  - – Sterile occlusive dressing
  - – Luer locks
  - – Scalpel: no. 11 blade
  - – Dilator
  - – Biopatch
  - – Fasteners
  - – Suture
  - – Needle driver

■ **Patient/scanner position**

- IJ
  - ○ Place patient supine Trendelenburg position (15–20°)
  - ○ Head turned contralateral
  - ○ Scanner at head of bed
  - ○ Probe marker toward scanner's left
- Subclavian
  - ○ Scanner standing to the side of selected site
  - ○ Patient supine
  - ○ Probe marker toward scanner's left
- Femoral
  - ○ Scanner at site selected
  - ○ Patient supine
  - ○ Leg slightly flexed and rotated outward
  - ○ Probe marker toward scanner's left

■ **Central venous catheter—US-guided Seldinger technique**

- Access of subclavian and femoral vein procedural technique is the same for IJ EXCEPT position of scanner, patient, vessel, and anatomy.

■ **Internal jugular vein cannulation**

- Collect all medical supplies.
- Ensure patient is on the monitor with frequent vital signs and cardiac monitoring.

- Place nonsterile probe on vessel of interest using small amount of gel.
- Identify vascular structures in short axis.
- Differentiate between artery, vein and nerve utilizing compression, pulsation, and color Doppler.
- Scan entirety of the vessel to evaluate for thrombus.
- Prepare sterile field.
- Gown and glove in sterile fashion.
- Place sterile towels and drape.
- Apply sterile gel and cover on probe, secure with supplied rubber bands.
- Apply sterile ultrasound gel to probe cover, re-locate vessel.
- Prepare and inject local anesthetic in wheel like fashion.
- Pre-flush with sterile normal saline each lumen of the CVC, make sure all clamps are secured on each lumen prior to access.
- Leave brown port without luer lock as this is where the guide wire will exit.
- Maintain constant gentle negative pressure on syringe while inserting 18G introducer needle attached to 10 mL syringe at a 45° angle tracking the needle tip.
- Tenting of the vessel should be visualized and the needle tip in the vessel with blood pulled back into syringe.
- Remove syringe from introducer needle, blood should ooze from the needle.
- Insert J-tip guidewire into needle port and rotate probe into longitudinal plane to confirm placement within the vein.
- Remove introducer needle while maintaining constant contact with the guidewire.
- Make small skin nick with no.11 blade scalpel, careful to avoid cutting guidewire.
- Insert dilator over guidewire and slowly rotate in clockwise motion.
- Remove dilator, maintain control of guidewire.
- Advance the triple lumen catheter over the guidewire, again constant contact with the guidewire at all times is critical.
- Remove the guidewire from the brown port after central line has been fully advanced.
- Apply luer lock to brown port, ensure blood return and flush each port with sterile normal saline.
- Apply Biopatch or antibacterial-impregnated sterile dressing.
- Suture the skin to the fasteners on the catheter.
- Clean site with Chloraprep or other antiseptic solution as necessary.
- Apply sterile occlusive dressing.
- Order STAT chest x-ray for line placement confirmation and clearance to utilize.

## PEARLS AND PITFALLS

- Vessel access contraindication is a thrombosis identified in the vein.

- Always evaluate for pneumothorax post procedure identifying evidence of lung sliding.

- Slowly advance into the vessel tilting the probe to track the needle tip.

- Always have a hand on the guidewire while it is inserted into the vein.

- Venous thrombosis appears as a variable echogenicity within lumen of vein.

- Repetition is key. Always perform the steps in the same order to ensure you do not miss a step when it matters most.

## BIBLIOGRAPHY


Avila, J. (2022, June). *Ultrasound-guided peripheral IV access*. Core Ultrasound. https://coreultrasound.com/ultrasound-guided-peripheral-iv-access/

Ferrada, P. (2020a, June). *How to do internal jugular vein cannulation, ultrasound-guided*. Merck Manuals Professional Version. https://www.merckmanuals.com/professional/critical-care-medicine/how-to-do-central-vascular-procedures/how-to-do-internal-jugular-vein-cannulation,-ultrasound-guided

Ferrada, P. (2020b, June). *How to do femoral vein cannulation, ultrasound-guided*. Merck Manuals Professional Version. https://www.merckmanuals.com/professional/critical-care-medicine/how-to-do-central-vascular-procedures/how-to-do-femoral-vein-cannulation,-ultrasound-guided

Franco-Sadud, R., Schnobrich, D., Mathews, B. K., Candotti, C., Abdel-Ghani, S., Perez, M. G., Rodgers, S. C., Mader, M. J., Haro, E. K., Dancel, R., Cho, J., Grikis, L., Lucas, B. P., the SHM Point-of-care Ultrasound Task Force, & Soni, N. J. (2019). Recommendations on the use of ultrasound guidance for central and peripheral vascular access in adults: A position statement of the society of hospital medicine. *Journal of Hospital Medicine* 14(9), E1–E22. https://www.ncbi.nlm.nih.gov/pmc/articles/PMC10193861/

Genobaga, S., Cleek, J., & Lee, V. Ultrasound-guided central line placement made easy: Step-by-step guide. In V. Dinh (Ed.), POCUS101. https://www.pocus101.com/ultrasound-guided-central-line-placement-made-easy-step-by-step-guide/

Heffner, A. C., & Androes, M. P. (2023, June). Central venous access in adults: General principles of placement. *UpToDate*. https://www.uptodate.com/contents/central-venous-access-in-adults-general-principles

Lee, V., & Kempf, H. Ultrasound-guided peripheral IV insertion, placement, and access made easy. In V. Dinh (Ed.), POCUS101. https://www.pocus101.com/ultrasound-guided-peripheral-iv-insertion-placement-and-access-made-easy/

# PARACENTESIS, PERICARDIOCENTESIS, ARTHROCENTESIS, THORACENTESIS

Ari Chaskes

## INTRODUCTION

- Provides diagnostic and therapeutic intervention
- Standard of care for procedural guidance as supported by multiple organizations
- Cardiac tamponade is known to be present in 67% of pulseless electrical activity (PEA) cardiac arrests and is treatable.
- Success rate of 97% for point-of-care ultrasound (POCUS) guided pericardiocentesis
- Decreases failed procedure attempts and traumatic pneumothorax (odds ratio 0.3–0.8)
- Arthrocentesis of the shoulder with POCUS improves success rates from 61% to 89%
- In knee arthrocentesis, POCUS needle placement improves from 78% to 96%

See Tables 17.1 and 17.2 for indications and differentials.

**Table 17.1** Indications

| Abominable pain, distention, peritoneal tenderness | Chest pain, jugular vein distension | Dyspnea, tachypnea, fever, cough |
|---|---|---|
| Hemodynamic instability | Trauma | Joint pain, swelling, effusion |

**Table 17.2** Differentials

| • Cardiac tamponade<br>• ACS<br>• AAA | • Pericardial effusion<br>• Edema, pneumonia<br>• ARDS<br>• COVID-19<br>• Mass | • Septic<br>• Joint/arthritis | • Gout<br>• Pseudogout |
|---|---|---|---|
| • Ascites<br>• Bowel perforation<br>• Bowel obstruction pancreatitis<br>• Cholecystitis<br>• Appendicitis | • Spontaneous bacterial peritonitis<br>• Crohn's<br>• Ulcerative colitis | • Solid organ injury | • Pregnancy |

AAA, abdominal aortic aneurysm; ACS, acute coronary syndrome; ARDS, acute respiratory distress syndrome; COVID-19, coronavirus disease 2019

## IMAGE ACQUISITION

- **Probe**
  - Curvilinear: ideal for abdominal and paracentesis due to its deeper penetration
  - Linear: best for thoracentesis
  - Phased array: preferred for cardiac and pericardiocentesis due to its ability to visualize deeper structures
- **Hand placement**
  - Lung and joint view: hold like a pencil
  - Cardiac subcostal view: hold like a pencil
  - Abdominal view: "cupping" probe with knuckles toward the bed or hold like a pencil
- **Technique**
  - Always maintain proper orientation

> **PRO TIP**
>
> Cardiac preset changes orientation marker to right side of screen.

- All windows should be visualized in transverse and longitudinal planes.
- Use Doppler mode and high-frequency probe to ensure areas of vasculature.
- Identify insertion site by area of largest fluid collection with adequate distance from organs and vessels.

## ANATOMY/IMAGES

See Figures 17.1 and 17.2 for images depicting abdominal anatomy and arthrocentesis procedure of the left hip.

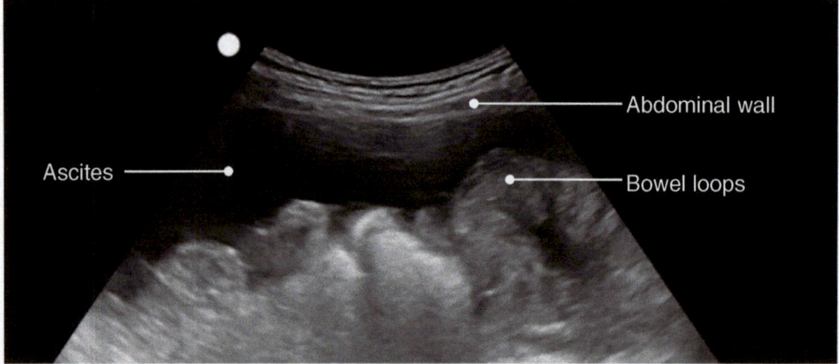


**Figure 17.1.** Abdominal anatomy with ascites bowel floating in free fluid.

*Source:* Image courtesy of SonoSim US-Guided Paracentesis.

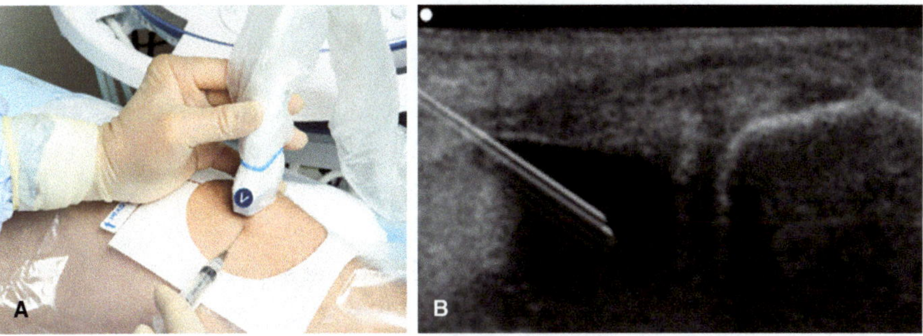

**Figure 17.2.** Arthrocentesis procedure. (A) Proper position. (B) US guided needle placement.

*Source*: Images courtesy of SonoSim, Musculoskeletal: Core Clinical, 2024.

## INTERPRETATION

- Black fluid (anechoic) surrounding or inside a hyperechoic organ capsule is free fluid/blood.
- Black, anechoic collection surrounding joint space is free fluid/effusion
- Anechoic collection surrounding bowel loops is ascites
- Lung tissue that appears to be floating in dark anechoic fluid is likely pleural effusion

See Table 17.3 for a description of procedural equipment.

**Table 17.3** Procedural Equipment

| Procedure | Equipment |
|---|---|
| Equipment for all procedures | • Sterile gloves/ probe cover/drapes/dressing<br>• Local anesthetic<br>• Various needles, syringes<br>• Chlorhexidine/iodine swabs<br>• Transducer of choice |
| Pericardiocentesis | • Probe: phased array<br>• ***Pro Tip: Change to linear probe for vascular assessment***<br>• Preset: cardiac<br>• 10 mL syringe, 16g–18 g needle<br>• Pigtail catheter (if placing pericardial drain)<br>• Arterial line kit for guidewire |
| Thoracentesis | • Probe: linear or phased array<br>• Preset: lung<br>• Paracentesis/thoracentesis tray<br>• Drainage bag<br>• Chest tube or pigtail dependent on size of effusion |
| Paracentesis | • Probe: curvilinear, linear, phased array<br>• Preset: abdominal/FAST<br>• Paracentesis/thoracentesis tray<br>• Drainage bottles |
| Arthrocentesis | • Probe: linear probe<br>• Preset: MSK<br>• Local anesthetic<br>• 18 g needle, 10 mL syringe |

FAST, focused assessment with sonography in trauma; MSK, musculoskeletal

## PATIENT/SCANNER POSITION

- **Pericardiocentesis**
  - Patient supine or semi-lateral decubitus, head of bed 30 to 45°
  - Scanner: same side as procedural site
- **Thoracentesis**
  - Patient
    - Position of comfort, seated on edge of bed, feet supported, torso leaning forward, arm crossed, supported on a table
    - Sitting position not tolerated: head of bed at 60 to 90°, lateral recumbent position
  - Scanner
    - Behind patient looking posterior to anterior
- **Paracentesis**
  - Patient
    - Supine, lateral decubitus, head of bed 30 to 45°
  - Scanner
    - Same side as procedural site
- **Joint Effusion**
  - Patient
    - Joint slightly flexed, supported, and fully relaxed
  - Scanner
    - Same side as procedural site

See Table 17.4 for information on site selection and Table 17.5 for summary of pathologic findings.

**Table 17.4** Site Selection

| Pericardiocentesis | Thoracentesis |
|---|---|
| • *Pro Tip: Obtain all cardiac views if able*<br>• Assess IVC collapsibility and diameter<br>• Subcostal view is best near xiphoid process and left costal margin<br>• *Contraindications*: None in an unstable patient. Relative include coagulopathy, low platelets, provider knowledge regarding chest anatomy | • *Pro Tip: Obtain a complete lung exam*<br>• Must identify diaphragm<br>• Identify space with largest distance from lung tissue, diaphragm, and organs during the entire respiratory cycle<br>• At minimum, a 1.5 cm depth of effusion must be visible for consideration<br>• *Contraindications*: coagulopathy disorders, bleeding disorders |
| **Paracentesis** | **Arthrocentesis** |
| • *Pro Tip: Obtain a FAST exam for complete abdominal evaluation*<br>• Use the window with the largest fluid collection and largest amount of distance between abdominal wall and bowel<br>• Lateral to rectus abdominis muscles and near aponeurosis | • *Pro Tip: linear probe for all MSK joints EXCEPT hip, consider curvilinear*<br>• Select affected joint, always scan contralateral side<br>• Window with the best view of the effusion<br>• Avoid windows with large vessels or nerves in the path of the needle |

*(continued)*

**Table 17.4** Site Selection (*continued*)

| Paracentesis | Arthrocentesis |
|---|---|
| • Use real-time or static images<br>• *Contraindications*: Coagulopathy, thrombocytopenia, thrombocytopathy, hyperfibrinolysis, extensive adhesions, abdominal scars, extensive abdominal surgery, hernia, ST cellulitis, advanced pregnancy, masses, organomegaly | • Familiarity with MSK anatomy is critical<br>• *Contraindications*: Overlying infection, cellulitis, multiple joint taps, recent surgery, recent trauma |

IVC, inferior vena cava; MSK, musculoskeletal; ST, soft tissue.

**Table 17.5** Summary of Pathologic Findings

| Condition | Ultrasound Findings |
|---|---|
| Cardiac tamponade | A pericardial effusion (larger size associated with tamponade), diastolic right ventricular collapse (specific), systolic right atrial collapse (sensitive), a noncollapsible IVC (sensitive), dilated IVC 97% sensitivity<br>***Pro Tips:***<br>• ***Effusion is positioned anterior to descending aorta***<br>• ***Epicardial fat pad is usually found only anteriorly*** |
| Pleural effusion | Identification of a hypoechoic or anechoic space surrounded by normal anatomic boundaries and lung tissue<br>May see "lung flapping" or "jellyfish sign"<br>***Pro Tips:***<br>• ***Effusion is positioned posterior to descending aorta***<br>• ***Always locate the diaphragm*** |
| Joint effusion | Collection of hypoechoic fluid that often sits near anatomic location of fat pad in different joints |
| Ascites | Anechoic fluid in the abdominal cavity surrounding loops of bowel, with or without debris and septations |

IVC, inferior vena cava

## PEARLS AND PITFALLS

- Always scan contralateral side for comparison
- Always use color Doppler to confirm presence of vascular structures using linear probe
- Position of patient at 30 to 45° improves fluid collection in the most dependent regions
- Consider prior surgeries that may alter fluid accumulation and anatomy
- Determine pleural effusion versus pericardial effusion based on location of fluid in relation to the aorta.
- The diaphragm will reside higher in a low tidal volume state in vented patients.
- Take no more than 6 L off initially to prevent flash pulmonary edema

## VIDEOS

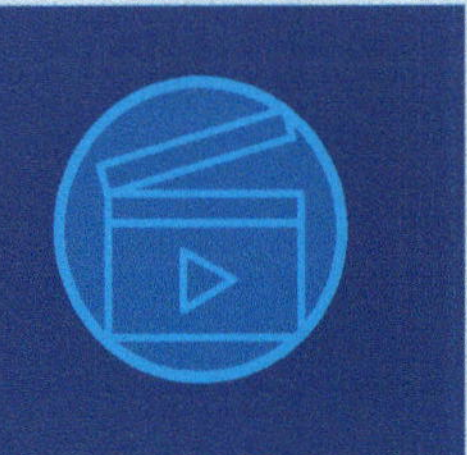

- Arthrocentesis
- Paracentesis
- Pericardiocentesis
- Pericardial Effusion
- Pleural Effusion—Thoracentesis
- Subxiphoid/Subcostal View
- Thoracentesis

**To access the videos, please go to the List of Videos in the front matter.**

## BIBLIOGRAPHY

Alerhand, S., Adrian, R. J., Long, B., & Avila, J. (2022). Pericardial tamponade: A comprehensive emergency medicine and echocardiography review. *American Journal of Emergency Medicine, 58*, 159–174. https://doi.org/10.1016/j.ajem.2022.05.001

American College of Emergency Physicians. (2023). *Ultrasound guidelines: Emergency, point-of-care, and clinical ultrasound guidelines in medicine.* https://www.acep.org/siteassets/sites/acep/media /ultrasound/pointofcareultrasound-guidelines.pdf

Bramante, R. M., & Harrison, C. W. (202, October 28). *Arthrocentesis.* American College of Emergency Physicians. https://www.acep.org/sonoguide/procedures/arthrocentesis

Getnet, W., Kebede, T., Atinafu, A., & Sultan, A. (2019). The value of ultrasound in characterizing and determining the etiology of ascites. *Ethiopian Journal of Health Sciences, 29*(3), 383–390. https://doi .org/10.4314/ejhs.v29i3.11

Lazaros, G., Vlachopoulos, C., Lazarou, E., & Tsioufis, K. (2021). New approaches to management of pericardial effusions. *Current Cardiology Reports, 23*(8), 106. https://doi.org/10.1007/s11886-021-01539-7

Poonja, Z., Ahn, J. S., & Kim, D. J. (2021). Just the facts: Ultrasound guidance for arthrocentesis. *Canadian Journal of Emergency Medicine, 23*(6), 737–739. https://doi.org/10.1007/s43678-021-00184-x

Shah, A., Barnes, R. M., Rocco, L. E., Robinson, C., Kubalak, S. W., Wahlquist, A. E., & Presley, B. C. (2023). Measuring success: A comparison of ultrasound and landmark guidance for knee arthrocentesis in a cadaver model. *American Journal of Emergency Medicine, 71*, 157–162. https://doi.org/10.1016/j.ajem .2023.06.044

Soni, N. J., Arntfield, R., & Kory, P. (2020). *Point-of-care ultrasound* (2nd ed.). Elsevier. Willner, D. A., & Grossman, S. A. (2024). Pericardiocentesis. In *StatPearls*. StatPearls Publishing. Copyright © 2024, StatPearls Publishing LLC.

# CHAPTER 18

# INCISION AND DRAINAGE

Meghan Petzy

## INTRODUCTION

- Soft tissue (ST) infections are among the top 20 diagnoses with highest number of treat and release visits (Avila, 2020).
- Differentiating between cellulitis, abscess, necrotizing fasciitis, and gas gangrene is a fundamental application of point-of-care-ultrasound (POCUS).
- POCUS, an extension of physical exam, provides accurate evaluation of differentials with 97% sensitivity and 83% specificity, respectively (Pastorino & Tavarez, 2023)
- POCUS changes management plans in about 50% of ST cases: incision and drainage (I&D) versus antibiotics alone (Ramirez-Schrempp et al., 2009)
- Detects nonradiopaque foreign bodies with sensitivity and specificity 96.7% to 100% (Soni et al., 2020)

See Tables 18.1 and 18.2 for indications and differentials.

**Table 18.1** Indications

| Warm, erythematous induration | Tender, swelling | Trauma |
|---|---|---|
| Diabetic wounds, ulcers | Skin lesions, rash | Area of purulence |

**Table 18.2** Differentials

| Abscess | Cellulitis | Necrotizing fasciitis | Foreign body |
|---|---|---|---|
| Pseudoaneurysm | Soft tissue mass, hematoma | Lymphadenitis | Malignancy |

## IMAGE ACQUISITION

- **Probe**
  - Linear
  - Curvilinear: deeper than 4 cm, large body habitus
- **Hand placement**
  - Hold like a pencil

■ **Technique**

- Preset: musculoskeletal (MSK) or ST
- Probe marker to scanner's left

**PRO TIP**

Use an adequate amount of gel to avoid the need for excessive pressure at the site of evaluation.

■ Scan the entire area of concern, including local areas with uninvolved anatomy to better appreciate normal versus abnormal findings.

- Compare to the contralateral side
- Tilt and fan in two planes (longitudinal and transverse)
  - ○ Allows for an estimate of the size of collection and visualization of potential blood vessels and other surrounding structures
- Gentle pressure may elicit movement of fluid providing more evidence of the presence of an abscess
- Use calipers to measure dimensions in two planes.
- Color or Doppler flow may be used if concern for vascular structure or pseudoaneurysm

## ANATOMY/IMAGES

See Figures 18.1 through 18.3 for images depicting normal ST, abscess with minor cobblestoning, and necrotizing fasciitis (hyperechoic flecks).

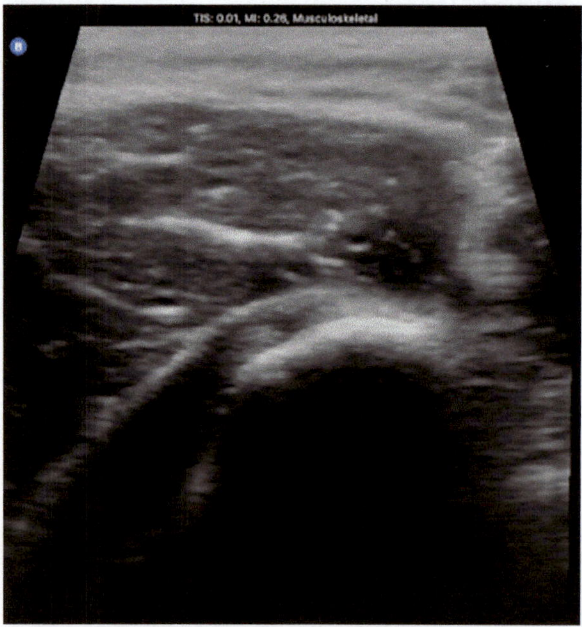


**Figure 18.1.** Normal soft tissue with muscle, tendon, and cortical line with bone shadow.
*Source:* Used with permission. Image courtesy of Dr. Kelli Craven.

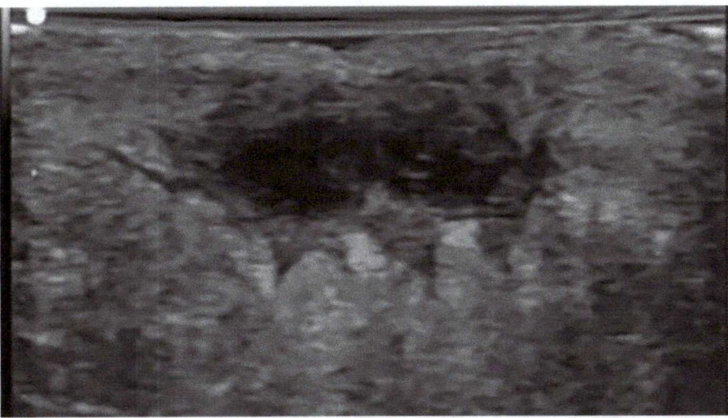

**Figure 18.2.** Abscess with mild cobblestoning.

*Source*: Image courtesy SonoSim, MSK, challenge cases, 2024, musculoskeletal-challenge-cases#_Q2FzZVR5c GU6NzgzZTI2MTItNGE2ZS00YTE4LTgxZDQtMmE1M2NiNmJmN2Vm.

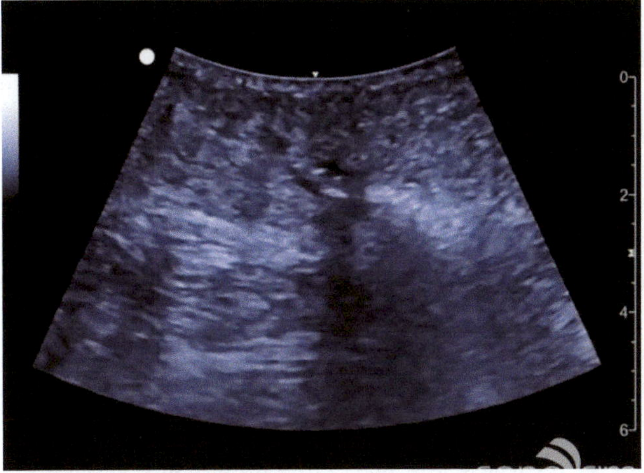

**Figure 18.3.** Necrotizing fasciitis (hyperechoic flecks, dirty shadowing, thick dermal tissues).

*Source*: Image courtesy of Sonosim, soft tissue case study, 2024, case-study-sft-0300/case-study/case-study-sft-0200.

## INTERPRETATION

See Table 18.3 for a summary of pathologic findings.

**Table 18.3** Summary of Pathologic Findings

| Condition | Ultrasound Findings |
| --- | --- |
| Cellulitis | Thick subcutaneous tissue, cobblestoning |
| Abscess | Anechoic/hyperechoic fluid collection, posterior acoustic enhancement, swirling with compression, hyperemia with color flow Doppler |
| Necrotizing fasciitis | STAFF: subcutaneous thickening, air, fascial fluid, air in soft tissues = pathognomonic |

## INCISION AND DRAINAGE PROCEDURE

■ **Equipment**
  - Linear transducer
  - Laceration tray
  - Iodine/chlorhexidine
  - No. 11 or No. 15 blade
  - Anesthetic of choice
  - Chux
  - 4 by 4 inch gauze
■ **US preset**
  - Vascular or ST
■ **Hand position**

  - Holding like an okay sign
■ **Procedure**
  - Confirm presence of an abscess
    ◦ Prepare the patient for I&D as indicated
    ◦ Measure the area of anechoic fluid
    ◦ Measure the depth from the surface to anechoic fluid
    ◦ Cleanse the skin with iodine/chlorhexidine
    ◦ Sterile drape as indicated
    ◦ Sterile or clean technique
    ◦ Anesthetize the area in a square-like pattern and at puncture site with a wheel
    ◦ Observe in real time while incising the abscess. Using proper blade, make an X on surface of skin for proper evacuation of fluid
    ◦ Use Q-tips or hemostat to break up loculations inside the abscess
  - Rescan postprocedure to evaluate for any remaining fluid collections denoted by pockets of anechoic fluid.

## PEARLS AND PITFALLS

■ Physical exam findings alone fail to differentiate between abscess, cellulitis, foreign body, and necrotizing fasciitis
■ Necrotizing fasciitis: a "do not" miss differential and potentially fatal bacterial infection
■ Color flow Doppler is valuable to identify vascular structures and avoid unnecessary, harmful I&D attempts
■ Water baths are an excellent medium to view the hand/digits
■ Cobblestoning is a nonspecific finding that can also represent subcutaneous edema
  - Clinical signs of infection needed to be attributed to cellulitis

■ Contraindications include large/deep abscesses, pulsatile masses, close proximity to vasculature, sensitive locations, foreign body

■ When to consult: abscesses of perineum, breasts, joints, neck, and/or vulva may be complicated and require alterations to treatment. Seek expert consultation (surgery, gynaecology, orthopedics, ENT)

## VIDEOS

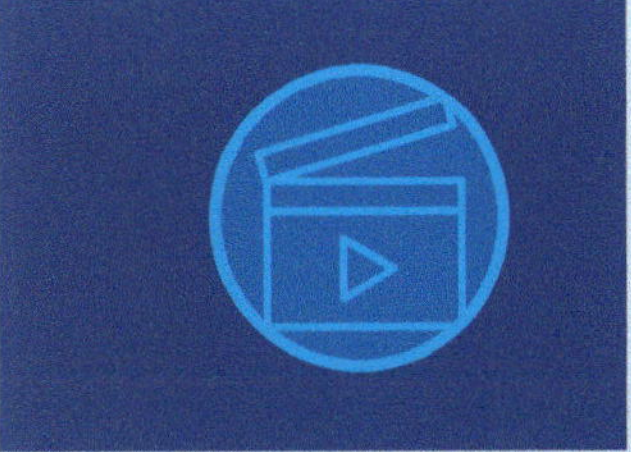

• **Identifying an Area for Draining an Abscess**

**To access the videos, please go to the List of Videos in the front matter.**

## BIBLIOGRAPHY

Avila, J. (2020, February 14). *Core Ultrasound: Cellulitis vs Abscess*. https://coreultrasound.com/cellulitis-vs-abscess/

Butterfly Network. (2023). *Ultrasound training videos for education: Butterfly network*. Retrieved July 1, 2023, from www.butterflynetwork.com/education

Pastorino, A., & Tavarez, M. (2023). Incision and Drainage. *Stat Pearls*.

Ramirez-Schrempp, D., Dorfman, D. H., Baker, W. E., & Liteplo, A. S. (2009). Ultrasound soft tissue applications in the pediatric emergency department. *Pediatric Emergency Care, 25*(1), 44–48. https://doi.org/10.1097/pec.0b013e318191d963

Soni, N. J., Arntfield, R., & Kory, P. (2020). *Point of care ultrasound* (2nd ed.). Elsevier.

Tayal, V. S., Hasan, N., Norton, H. J., & Tomaszewski, C. A. (2006). The effect of soft-tissue ultrasound on the management of cellulitis in the emergency department. *Academic Emergency Medicine, 13*(4), 384–388. https://doi.org/10.1197/j.aem.2005.11.074

Weiss, A. J., & Jiang, H. J. (2021, December). *Most frequent reasons for emergency department visits, 2018*. Most Frequent Reasons for Emergency Department Visits, 2018. https://hcup-us.ahrq.gov/reports/statbriefs/sb286-ED-Frequent-Conditions-2018.pdf

Wright, E., & Somwaru, B. (2020, December 14). *Pocus and soft tissue foreign bodies*. REBEL EM—Emergency Medicine Blog. https://rebelem.com/pocus-and-soft-tissue-foreign-bodies/

# CHAPTER 19

# LUMBAR PUNCTURE

Kelli Craven

## INTRODUCTION

- Spinal mapping with point of care ultrasound (POCUS) far exceeds physical exam alone.
- First demonstrated use in 1971
- POCUS is now the gold standard.
- Body mass index >30 decreases landmark identification, increasing failed attempts
- Ultrasound decreases failed attempts, traumatic taps, and needle redirection attempts
- Success rate > 95% with the use of US (Soni et al., 2020)
- Failure rate 19% using landmarks alone (Soni et al., 2020)
- Improved patient outcomes, less pain, less procedure time, and improved patient satisfaction scores

See Tables 19.1 and 19.2 for indications and differentials.

**Table 19.1** Indications

| AMS | Headache/neck stiffness | Fever/prodromal symptoms |
|---|---|---|
| Upper respiratory symptoms | Obesity | PE + screening for Meningitis |

AMS, altered mental status; PE, physical exam

**Table 19.2** Differentials

| Meningitis | URI | Mono |
|---|---|---|
| CVA/TIA | Hypoglycemia | AMS<br>Altered mental status mimickers (e.g., alcohol intoxication) |

AMS, altered mental status; CVA, cerebrovascular accident; TIA, transient ischemic attack; URI, upper respiratory infection

## IMAGE ACQUISITION

- **Probe**
  - Linear probe (high frequency) for thin or pediatric patients
  - Curvilinear probe (low frequency) for obese or deep lumbar spaces.

- **Hand placement**
  - "Okay" sign
- **Technique**
  - Find the L4 space by placing hand on the posterior superior iliac crests and aligning the thumbs pointing toward the spine—where the thumbs meet is usually L4. Mark with a skin marker then place the probe in transverse position on the location to identify the L4 spinous process.
  - Count the spinous processes up and down to map out L2–L5 by sliding the probe up and down.
  - Then, at L4, the probe is placed again; place the probe in a longitudinal position to identify the interspinous space between L4 and L5. Use dotted lines to mark this position, essentially making a cross with the dotted lines.
  - L4 has the largest interspinous space and is thus the best site for the procedure selection. However, L2–L5 may be considered

See Figure 19.1 for normal anatomy and spinal mapping.

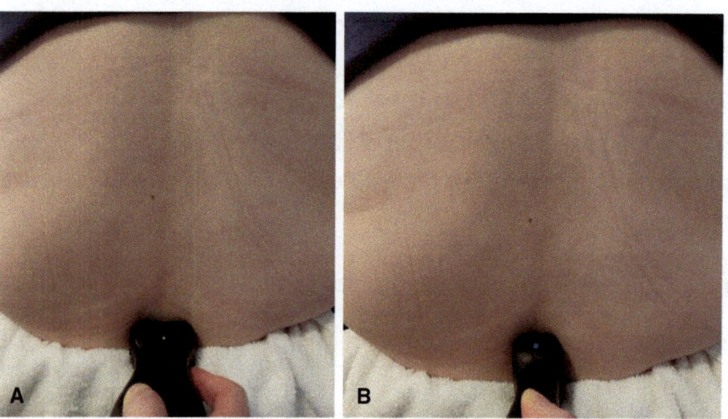

**Figure 19.1.** Normal anatomy and spinal mapping. (A) Transverse. (B) Longitudinal.
*Source*: Used with permission. Image courtesy of Dr. Kelli Craven.

## INTERPRETATION

- Cortical line is always hyperechoic in appearance and adjacent to the interspinous space
- Spinous process shadow is always hypoechoic
- On a longitudinal paramedian view, the ligamentum flavum-dura complex appears as a single or double hyperechoic line depending on resolution settings. Ligamentum flavum may appear as a hyperechoic line between the lamina.
- Measure the distance between the skin and the ligamentum flavum using a longitudinal paramedian view.
- This measurement helps determine the ideal needle depth, reducing the risk of false passes or traumatic taps.

## PROCEDURE

■ **Equipment**
- Lumbar puncture (LP)kit
- Gloves
- Ultrasound (US) gel
- Linear probe
- Skin marker
- Lidocaine
- Sterile drape
- Sterile gloves
- Betadine and or chlorhexidine swabs for cleansing the skin

■ **Patient/scanner position**
- It is most beneficial to have the patient sitting upright for spinal mapping.
- Patient sitting upright 90° with leg dangling off bed and leaning over a small table
- Have the patient round out the back as much as possible.
- Patient may also be positioned in a left lateral decubitus position with knees drawn into chest and rounding out the back as much as possible.
- Iliac crest is used as the landmark to place hands with thumb pointing medially toward the spine to align with L4
- Ultrasound always in line of site to avoid off-axis scanning and frequent head turning

■ **Site selection**
- L2–L4
- L4 is ideal

See Table 19.3 for a summary of imaging findings.

**Table 19.3** Summary of Imaging Findings

| Condition | Ultrasound Findings |
|---|---|
| Spinous process | Hyperechoic with shadowing |
| Ligamentum flavum | A small hyperechoic line between lamina |
| Interspinous process | Between two spinous process, isoechoic |
| Lamina | Hyperechoic lines beneath erector spinae |
| Erector spinae | Muscle appearing bundle above lamina |
| Posterior longitudinal ligament | Anterior to lamina, hyperechoic |

## PEARLS AND PITFALLS

■ Take care not to confuse the lamina for spinous processes. The erector spinae muscle should be visible just above the lamina.

- Ligamentum flavum should be measured in the longitudinal paramedian position for accurate depth from the skin.

## BIBLIOGRAPHY

Soni, N. J., Arntfield, R., & Kory, P. (2020). *Point-of-care ultrasound* (2nd ed.). Elsevier.

Soni, N. J., Franco-Sadud, R., Schnobrich, D., Dancel, R., Tierney, D. M., Salame, G., Restrepo, M. I., & McHardy, P. (2016). Ultrasound guidance for lumbar puncture. *Neurology: Clinical Practice*, 6(4), 358–368. https://doi.org/10.1212/CPJ.0000000000000265

# CHAPTER 20

# BLADDER ASPIRATION

Wesley Davis

## INTRODUCTION

- Used to obtain sterile urine sample directly from bladder or to relieve urinary retention when catheterization not possible or contraindicated
- Performed in pediatric patients, can also be used in adults in specific clinical situations
- Point-of-care ultrasound (POCUS) improves safety and accuracy of bladder aspiration by visualization of the bladder and surrounding structures.
- Ultrasound guidance minimizes the risk of complications such as bowel perforation or aspiration of the wrong structure and ensures the bladder is adequately filled before the procedure.

See Tables 20.1 and 20.2 for indications and differentials.

**Table 20.1** Indications

| | |
| --- | --- |
| Bladder fullness, abdominal fullness | Abdominal pain, nausea, constipation |
| Failed urethral catheterization or difficult catheterization | Fever, dysuria, urgency, frequency |

**Table 20.2** Differentials

| | | |
| --- | --- | --- |
| Mass | Trauma | Retention |
| Infection | Outlet obstruction | |

## IMAGE ACQUISITION

- **Probe**
  - Curvilinear or phased array
  - A linear probe may be used in pediatric patients or for very superficial imaging.
- **Hand placement**
  - The probe is usually held in the "pencil grip."
- **Technique**
  - The patient should be positioned supine with the abdomen exposed.
  - Apply a liberal amount of ultrasound gel to the lower abdomen, just above the pubic symphysis.

- Place the probe first in transverse view just above the pubic bone and angle/tilt it slightly caudally to visualize the bladder.

> **PRO TIP**
>
> Always image in longitudinal and transverse planes tilting and rocking the probe sweeping through the bladder and surrounding anatomy.

- Identify the bladder as an anechoic, oblong, structure and ensure that it is adequately filled (at least 2–4 cm deep in sagittal view).
- Measure the bladder volume
  - Volume (mL) = Width (cm) × Depth (cm) × Height (cm) × 0.52
- If the bladder is not sufficiently full, delay the procedure until the bladder volume increases.

## ANATOMY/IMAGES

See Figure 20.1 for an ultrasound image of a bladder.

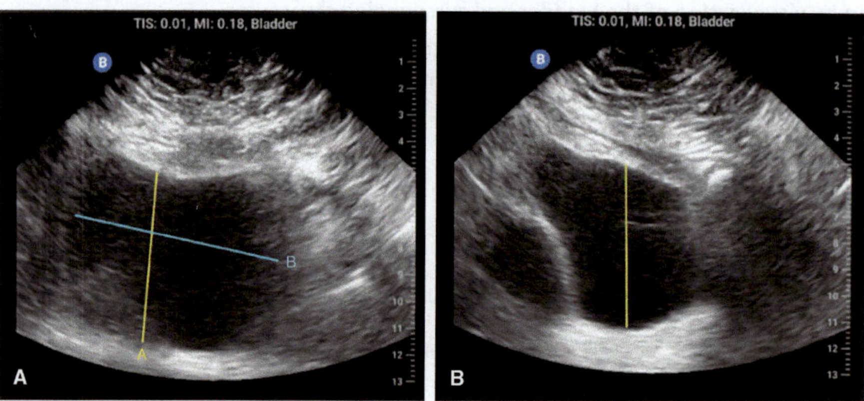


**Figure 20.1.** Ultrasound image of bladder. (A) Transverse bladder measurement. (B) Longitudinal bladder measurement.

*Source*: Used with permission. Image courtesy of Dr. Kelli Craven.

## INTERPRETATION

- Bladder appears as a round, oblong, or oval anechoic structure with well-defined walls.
- In a transverse view, it is positioned directly behind the pubic symphysis.
- Surrounding pelvic structures, including the uterus in females or the prostate in males, should also be identified to avoid inadvertent injury.
- Decreased bladder volume or thickening of the bladder wall may indicate chronic urinary retention or other underlying conditions.
- Pockets of echogenic material within the bladder may represent debris, blood clots, or less commonly, bladder stones.

- Accurate assessment of the bladder volume and identification of surrounding structures are critical before proceeding with bladder aspiration.
- The ultrasound image should show a well-distended bladder, free of significant debris or masses, to reduce the risk of complications.

## PROCEDURE

- **Equipment**
  - Sterile gloves and sterile field
  - Antiseptic solution for skin preparation
  - 22 gauge needle (long enough to reach the bladder but not too long to avoid penetrating beyond)
  - Syringe (10–20 mL) for aspiration
- **Patient/scanner position**
  - Patient should lie supine with the lower abdomen exposed.
  - The scanner stands to the side of the patient.
  - Ultrasound machine is positioned in line of site to prevent head turning and off-axis imaging.
- **Technique**
  - **Prepare the site:** Clean the skin over the lower abdomen with an antiseptic solution and drape the area to maintain a sterile field.
  - **Confirm the bladder location:** Use ultrasound to reconfirm the bladder's position and measure its depth.
  - **Needle insertion:** With real-time ultrasound guidance, insert the needle at a 10 to 20° angle caudally, directing it toward the bladder's center.
  - **Aspiration:** Advance the needle into the bladder lumen and aspirate urine into the syringe. Withdraw the needle once an adequate sample is obtained.
  - **Postprocedure:** Apply pressure to the site and monitor the patient for any signs of discomfort or complications.
- **Contraindications**
  - Recent abdominal/pelvic surgery or trauma
  - Bladder mass or known carcinoma
  - Coagulopathy disorders
  - Overlying skin infection/lesions

See Table 20.3 for a summary of pathologic findings.

**Table 20.3** Summary of Pathologic Findings

| Condition | Ultrasound Findings |
| --- | --- |
| Acute urinary retention | Enlarged, distended bladder |
| Bladder wall thickening | Hypoechoic or thickened bladder wall |
| Debris or blood clots in bladder | Echogenic material within the bladder lumen |
| Bladder stones | Hyperechoic focus with posterior shadowing |
| Uterine or prostate hypertrophy | Enlargement of adjacent structures, potentially compressing the bladder |

## PEARLS AND PITFALLS

- Always confirm the bladder is adequately filled before proceeding with aspiration.
- Use color Doppler to avoid puncturing any vessels that might be present near the bladder.
- Ensure proper needle alignment under ultrasound guidance to avoid penetrating too deeply or missing the bladder.
- Aspiration of an empty or inadequately filled bladder can lead to unsuccessful attempts and increase the risk of injury.
- Failure to maintain a sterile field can introduce infection, leading to complications such as bladder or abdominal wall abscess.
- Misidentification of the bladder or surrounding structures could result in accidental puncture of the bowel or blood vessels.

## BIBLIOGRAPHY

Fowler, G. C., & Lefevre, N. (2020). Emergency department, hospitalist, and office ultrasound (POCUS). In G. C. Fowler (Ed.), *Pfenninger and Fowler's procedures for primary care* (4th ed., pp. 1408–1438). Elsevier.

Nickels, L. C., & Duran-Gehring, P. (2023). Emergency ultrasound. In J. A. Marx, R. S. Hockberger, & R. M. Walls (Eds.), *Rosen's emergency medicine: Concepts and clinical practice* (10th ed.). Elsevier.

Werner, H., & Levy, J. (2011). Procedural applications of bedside emergency ultrasound. *Clinical Pediatric Emergency Medicine, 12*(1), 43–52. https://doi.org/10.1016/j.cpem.2010.12.003

# CHAPTER 21

# NERVE AND HEMATOMA BLOCKS

Juan M. Gonzalez

## INTRODUCTION

- Point-of-care ultrasound (POCUS) can guide single-point injections as a primary or adjunct therapy to reduce pain and improve patient comfort during emergency procedures.

- Injection of anesthesia near the nerves can be helpful to achieve pain reduction in any clinical setting when implemented as part of a comprehensive multimodal analgesia plan.

- POCUS-guided nerve blocks provide effective analgesia in procedures involving the neck and upper and lower extremities, reducing the need for systemic opioids or moderate sedation during fracture reduction.

- Hematoma blocks are a simpler alternative to nerve blocks for distal radius fractures and are particularly useful when nerve blocks are contraindicated. Use of a hematoma block to inject anesthetics shows similar efficacy to direct nerve blocks in patients with distal radial fractures (Abbasi et al., 2023)

- Nerve blocks typically take longer to achieve when compared to hematoma blocks, which are less complicated, however, there is no statistically significant increase in length of stays in the ED for patients receiving nerve blocks ($p = .313$) (Abbasi et al., 2023)

See Tables 21.1 and 21.2 for indications and differentials.

**Table 21.1** Indications

| Trauma, extremity deformity | Wound repair | Extensive wound debridement |
|---|---|---|
| Hematoma, abscess, infection | Joint deformity | Alternative to procedural sedation |

**Table 21.2** Differentials

| Fracture | Dislocation | Abscess |
|---|---|---|
| Laceration | Extensive wound repairs | Subluxation |

## IMAGE ACQUISITION

- **Probe:** high frequency, linear transducer (5–15 MHz)
- **Preset:** nerve
- **Hand position:** the "okay" sign is traditional hand placement to hold ultrasound for most scans

## TECHNIQUE

- Always maintain proper position of probe indicator to determine proper planes and anatomical position
- Indicator cephalad in long axis or performing the procedure in plane
- Indicator toward scanner's left in short-axis view or performing the procedure off-plane
- Short-axis (transverse) scanning provides a cross-sectional view of nerves, while long-axis (sagittal) scanning helps track needle movement during injection. Short axis or the transverse plane is preferred for nerve assessment.

## ANATOMY/IMAGES

See Figures 21.1 through 21.4 for images depicting brachial plexus, median nerve, femoral nerve, and posterior tibial nerve (PTN).

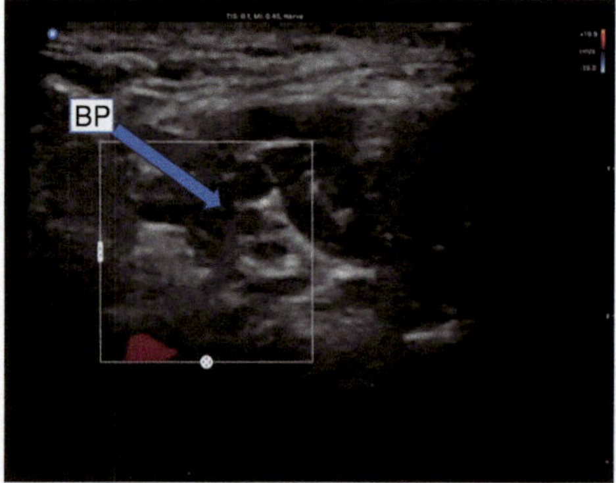


**Figure 21.1.** Brachial plexus.

*Note:* Anechoic structures, without any pulsation with the use of Doppler.

*Source:* Image by Juan M Gonzalez. Used with permission.

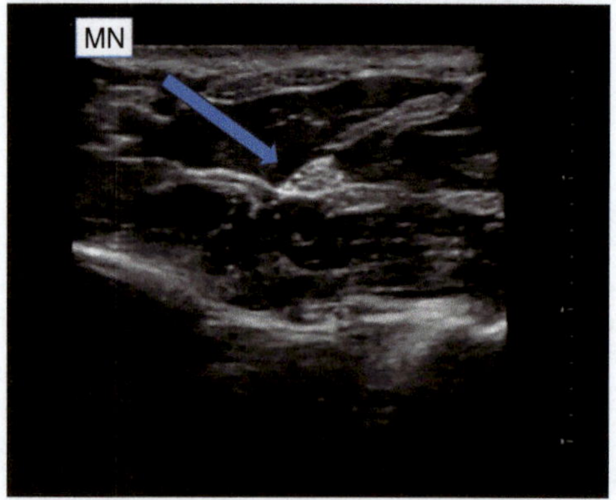


**Figure 21.2.** Median nerve.

*Source:* Image by Juan M Gonzalez. Used with permission.

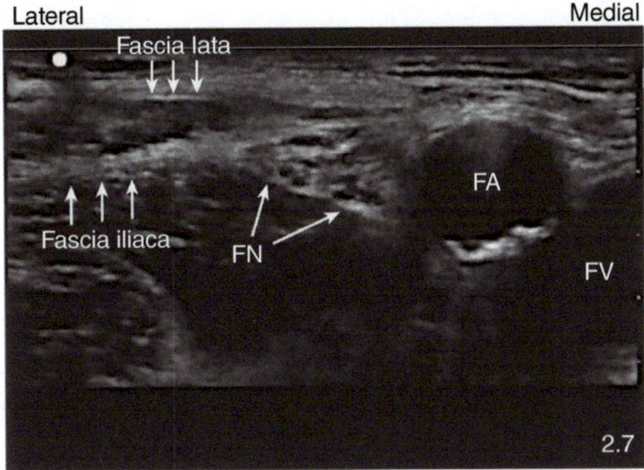


**Figure 21.3.** Femoral nerve.

*Source:* From Nagdev, A., LeVine, S., & Mantuani, D. (2020). Peripheral nerve blocks. In Nilam J. Soni, Robert Arntfield, & Pierre Kory (Eds.), *Point of care ultrasound* (2nd ed., pp. 389–404.e4) [e Book]. Elsevier, and used with permission from Elsevier, Inc.

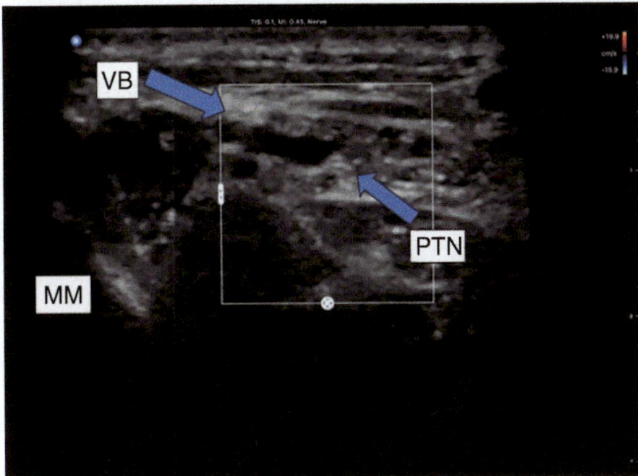


**Figure 21.4.** Posterior tibial nerve (PTN). Medial malleolus (MM), vascular bundle (VB).

*Source:* Image by Juan M Gonzalez. Used with permission.

## INTERPRETATION

- Nerves have a "honeycomb" appearance due to hyperechoic fascicles surrounded by hypoechoic connective tissue. Nerves appear honeycomb-like in nature.

- Brachial plexus appears as three circular structures with hypoechoic centers, may be confused with vasculature.

- Use color Doppler to rule out vascular structures.

- Hematomas appear as anechoic or hypoechoic fluid collections near fractured bone edges. Hematoma will appear near the interruption of the continuity of the bone and appears anechoic.

## PROCEDURE

### ■ Equipment

- Place the patient on telemetry monitoring and pulse ox for block procedures.
- Prep the skin with chlorhexidine or a similar solution.
- Sterile transducer sheath cover
- Syringe (control syringe is preferred)
- Needle (selection varies but usually from 25 to 30 G preferred)
- Lidocaine 1% to 2% generally used and recommended (max dose 4 mg/kg) with a duration of action of 1.5 to 2 hours.
- For prolonged analgesia (4 to 8 hours.), bupivacaine (0.25%–0.5%) can be used, but note the higher toxicity risk (max dose 3 mg/kg).
- Procedure can be done in-plane or off-plane.
- For distal radial fractures, as an alternative to a traditional nerve block, a hematoma block can be completed. The clinician, using US-guided injections, injects lidocaine directly into the hematoma.

---

**PRO TIP**

Utilize off access needle injection to verify needle position injecting a small amount of anesthetic while advancing towards the nerve bundle creating hydro-dissection of tissue allowing anesthetic to then be fully injected "bathing" or surrounding the nerve bundle.

---

### ■ Patient/scanner position

- US in line of vision on the opposite side to minimize head movement with the procedure and improve ergonomics
- Patient may be supine or prone.

### ■ Site selection

See Figures 21.5 through 21.7 for depictions of hematoma block for distal radial fracture reduction, supraclavicular brachial plexus nerve block, and in-plane approach for PTN block.

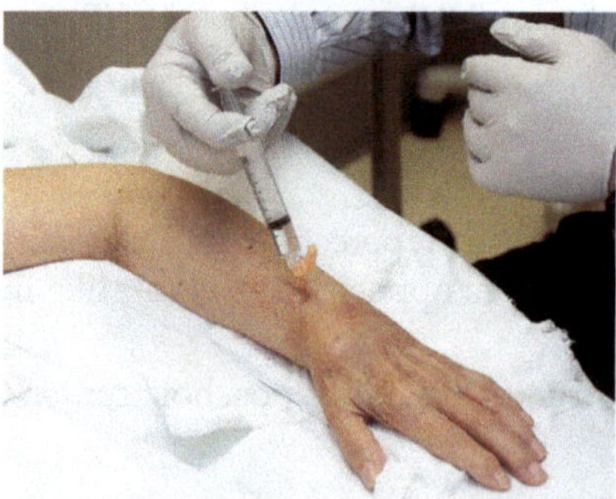

**Figure 21.5.** Hematoma block for distal radial fracture reduction.

*Source:* From McGee, D. L. (2019). Local and topical anesthesia. In James R. Roberts (Ed.), *Roberts and Hedges' clinical procedures in emergency medicine and acute care* (7th ed., pp. 523–544.e3) [e-book]. Elsevier, and used with permission from Elsevier, Inc.

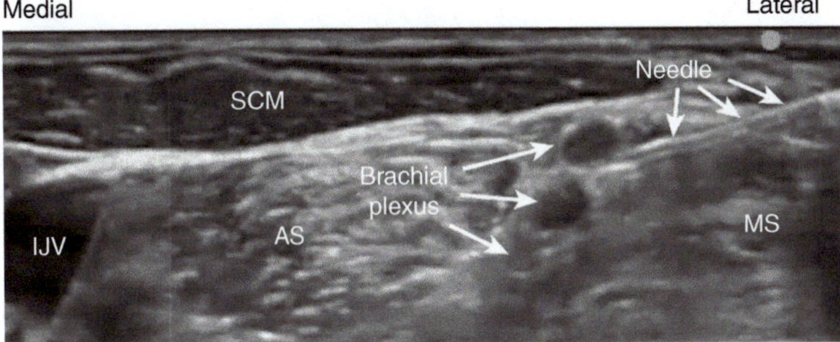



**Figure 21.6.** Supraclavicular brachial plexus nerve block.

*Source:* From Nagdev, A., LeVine, S., & Mantuani, D. (2020). Peripheral nerve blocks. In Nilam J Soni, Robert Arntfield, & Pierre Kory (Eds.), *Point of care ultrasound* (2nd ed., pp. 389–404.e4) [e Book]. Elsevier, and used with permission from Elsevier, Inc.

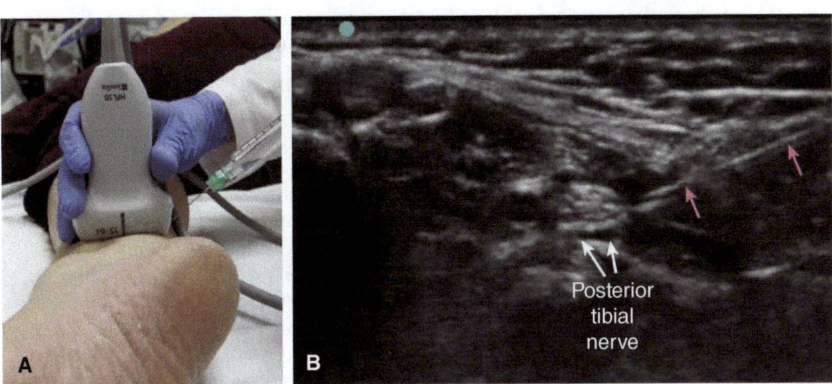



**Figure 21.7.** In-plane approach for posterior tibial nerve block.

*Source:* From Nagdev, A., LeVine, S., & Mantuani, D. (2020). Peripheral nerve blocks. In Nilam J Soni, Robert Arntfield, & Pierre Kory (Eds.), *Point of care ultrasound* (2nd ed., pp. 389–404.e4) [e Book]. Elsevier, and used with permission from Elsevier, Inc.

See Table 21.3 for a summary of ultrasound findings.

## Table 21.3 Summary of Ultrasound Findings

| Condition | Ultrasound Findings |
| --- | --- |
| Hematoma block | Anechoic collection near interrupted bone which appears hyperechoic with acoustic shadow. Inject anesthetic to this area. |
| Brachial plexus nerve block | Hyperechoic circular structures with anechoic center. No color pulsation with doppler. Inject anesthetic near the area but not inside the nerve. |
| Median nerve block | Hyperechoic honeycomb appearance. Inject the anesthesia near the nerve but not inside the nerve. |
| Femoral nerve block | Hyperechoic, honeycomb appearance. Nerve is lateral to femoral artery and vein (from lateral to medial → Nerve, artery → vein). Inject anesthesia near the nerve but not inside the nerve. |
| Posterior tibial block | Hyperechoic structure medial to the malleolus. Vascular bundle can be seen medially to the nerve. Inject anesthetic near but not inside the nerve. |

## PEARLS AND PITFALLS

- Patients should be neurologically intact and able to follow commands.
- A nerve block in compartment syndrome may mask progression.
- Although rare, peripheral nerve injury has been reported from 0% to 2.2% with nerve blocks. To avoid or decrease this issue, place the needle tip close to the nerve but NOT in the nerve itself.
- Procedure is not recommended in patients with peripheral neuropathy and should be interrupted if the patient develops worsening pain or new paresthesia.
- Review signs and symptoms of Local Anesthetic Systemic Toxicity (LAST) in case of accidental injection into the vessel.
  - Tongue numbness, dizziness, muscle twitching, decreased level of consciousness, seizures, and cardiovascular depression.
- In a situation where bupivacaine has been accidentally injected into the vessel, hyperlipophilic solution (20% intralipid, 1.5 mL/kg bolus should be given with continuous infusion at 0.25 mL/kg/min) and consult anesthesia.

## BIBLIOGRAPHY

Abbasi, S., Garjani, N., Mahshidfar, B., Farsi, D., Mofidi, M., Hafezimoghadam, P., Rezai, M., & Javan, A. (2023). Comparative study of radial and median nerve blocks with hematoma block under ultrasound guide in distal radius fracture reduction: A randomized clinical trial. *Medical Journal of The Islamic Republic of Iran, 37*(1), 886–891. https://doi.org/10.47176/mjiri.37.113

Maga, J., Missair, A., Visan, A., Kaplan, L., Gutierrez, J. F., Jain, A. R., & Gebhard, R. E. (2015). Comparison of outside versus inside brachial plexus sheath injection for ultrasound-guided interscalene nerve blocks. *Journal of Ultrasound in Medicine, 35*(2), 279–285. https://doi.org/10.7863/ultra.15.01059

Nagdev, A., McCarthy, C., & Martin, D. A. (2020). Nerve blocks. In J. P. McGahan, Schick, M. A., & L. D. Mills (Eds.), *Fundamentals of emergency ultrasound* (3rd ed., pp. 357–373) [e-book]. Elsevier.

Soares, L. G., Brull, R., & Chan, V. W. (2008). Teaching an old block a new trick: Ultrasound-guided posterior tibial nerve block. *Acta Anaesthesiologica Scandinavica, 52*(3), 446–447. https://doi.org/10.1111/j.1399-6576.2007.01515.x

# CHAPTER 22

# FRACTURES AND JOINT REDUCTIONS

Juan M. Gonzalez

## INTRODUCTION

- Point-of-care ultrasound (POCUS) is helpful in identifying fractures in both adults and pediatrics.

- The cortical bone appears hyperechoic on ultrasound, enabling clinicians to rapidly assess fractures and bone integrity using POCUS.

- POCUS-guided nerve blocks can be used in long bone fractures (e.g., femur, humerus) to provide effective analgesia, reducing the need for systemic opioids or sedation.

- In pediatrics, the use of ultrasound to diagnose fractures was first used in 1988 for suspected clavicular fractures.

- POCUS has also been shown to be beneficial in the diagnosis of occult fractures, such as scaphoid or rib fractures, as an alternative to MRIs.

- With the use of POCUS, clinicians are able to evaluate for early callus progression and also bone union, which takes longer to show in traditional x-ray.

- The combined sensitivity and specificity of ultrasound for detecting upper limb fractures is 0.93 and 0.92, respectively ($I^2 = 54.7\%$ and $66.3\%$), and 0.83 and 0.93 ($I^2 = 90.1\%$ and $83.5\%$) for lower limb fractures.

- For pediatrics, POCUS has shown a sensitivity of 95.8% and specificity of 98.5% to detect adequate fracture reductions.

See Table 22.1 for indications and Table 22.2 for differentials.

**Table 22.1** Indications

| Trauma/injury | Pain | Redness, swelling |
|---|---|---|
| Hematoma | Deformity | Limited range of motion |

**Table 22.2** Differentials

| Fracture, occult fracture | Dislocation | Subluxation |
|---|---|---|

## IMAGE ACQUISITION

- **Probe**
  - High frequency, linear transducer (5-15 MHz) for superficial structures
  - Curvilinear transducer for deeper structures such as the femur which may have more tissue over the bone

- **Preset**
  - Musculoskeletal (MSK)
- **Hand placement**
  - Traditional hand placement

## TECHNIQUE

- Probe marker toward scanner's left for transverse plane
- Indicator should be cephalad when obtaining a long axis or performing the procedure in plane.
- A **longitudinal scan** provides the best view of cortical disruption, while a **transverse scan** helps assess displacement or step-off.
- Short axis or transverse plane is preferred to assess nerves.

## ANATOMY/IMAGES

See Figures 22.1 through 22.6 for a depiction of normal cortical presentation with hyperechoic cortex of bone with acoustic shadowing

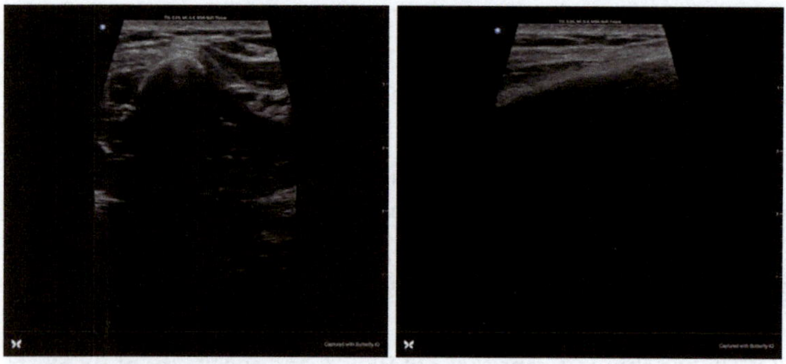

**Figure 22.1.** Normal radius, short and long axis.
*Source*: Image by Juan M. Gonzalez. Used with permission.

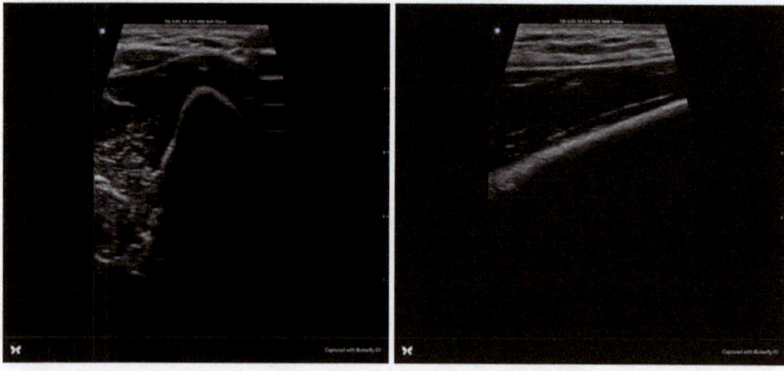

**Figure 22.2.** Normal ulna, short and long axis.
*Source*: Image by Juan M. Gonzalez, Used with permission.

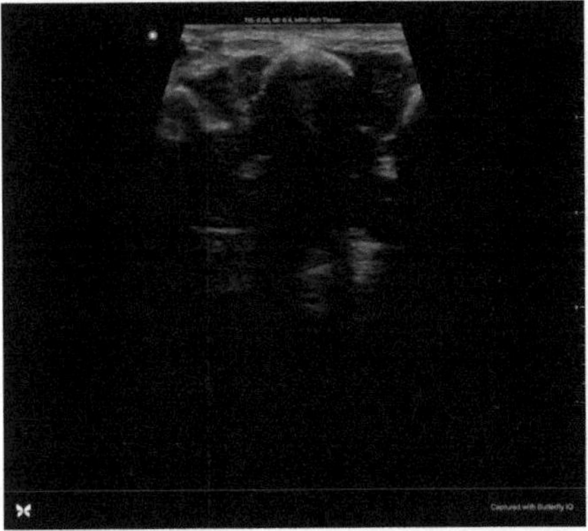

**Figure 22.3.** Normal carpal bones, short axis.
*Source*: Image by Juan M. Gonzalez. Used with permission.

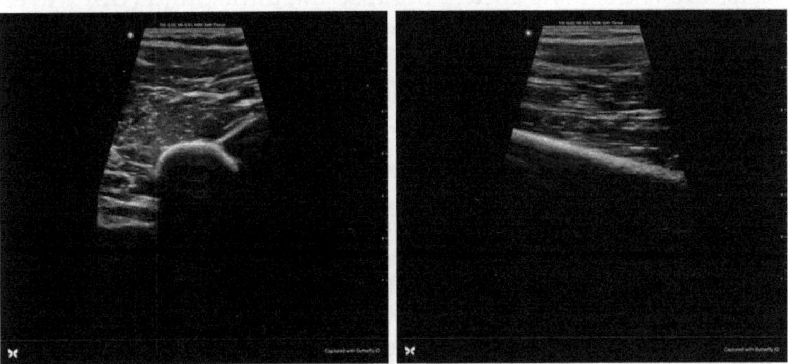

**Figure. 22.4.** Normal humerus, short and long axis.
*Source*: Image by Juan M. Gonzalez, Used with permission.

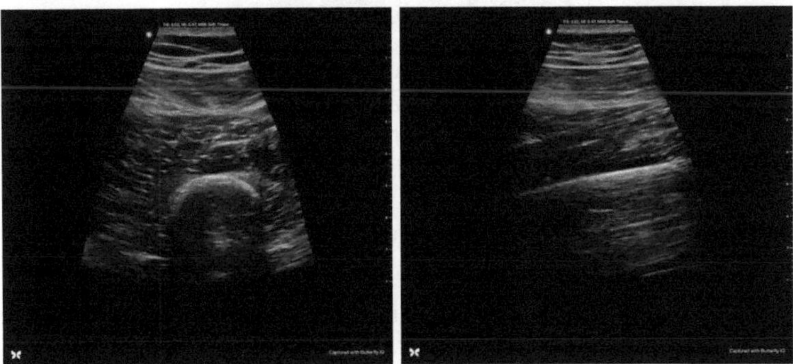

**Figure. 22.5.** Normal femur, short and long axis.
*Source*: Image by Juan M. Gonzalez. Used with permission.

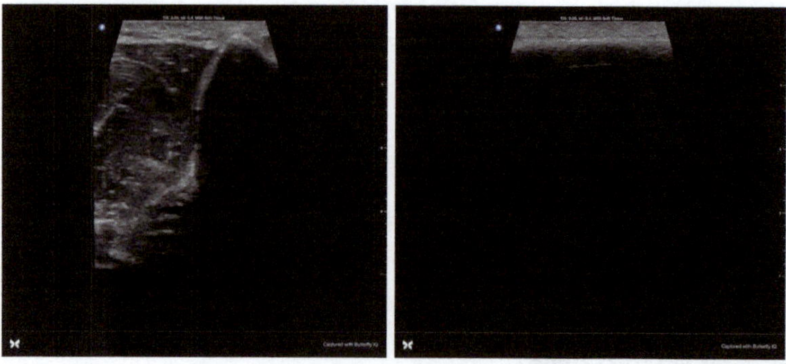

**Figure 22.6.** Normal tibia, short and long axis.

*Source*: Image by Juan M. Gonzalez. Used with permission.

## INTERPRETATION

- Hyperechoic structure is the bone cortex. Because the ultrasound (US) waves cannot penetrate bone, an acoustic shadow (anechoic) forms behind this hyperechoic structure.

See Figure 22.7 for an image depicting pediatric radial fracture and angulation.

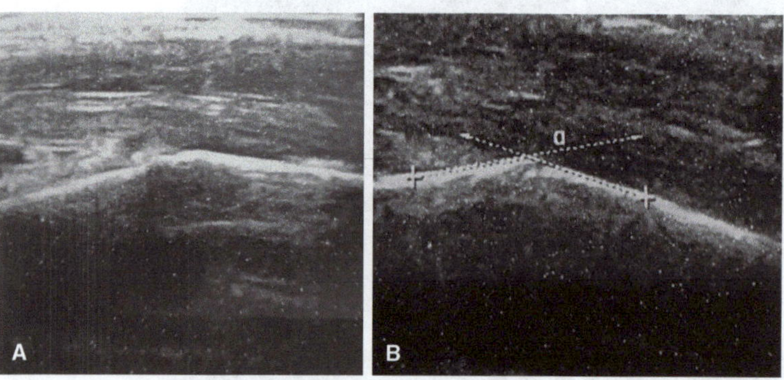

**Figure 22.7.** (A) Radial cortical "step-off" and (B) fracture angulation.

*Source*: From Şık, N., Öztürk, A., Koşay, M. C., Yılmaz, D., & Duman, M. (2021). Accuracy of point-of-care ultrasound for determining the adequacy of pediatric forearm fracture reductions. *The American Journal of Emergency Medicine*, *48*, 243–248. https://doi.org/10.1016/j.ajem.2021.05.021. Used with permission from Elsevier, Inc.

See Figure 22.8 for an image depicting distal radial fracture and postreduction assessment with POCUS.

See Figure 22.9 for an image depicting ultrasound used to assess humerus fracture, compared to x-ray.

## PEARLS AND PITFALLS

- POCUS is operator-dependent.
- Ensure you have proper training related to MSK ultrasound techniques and seek feedback from experienced scanners.

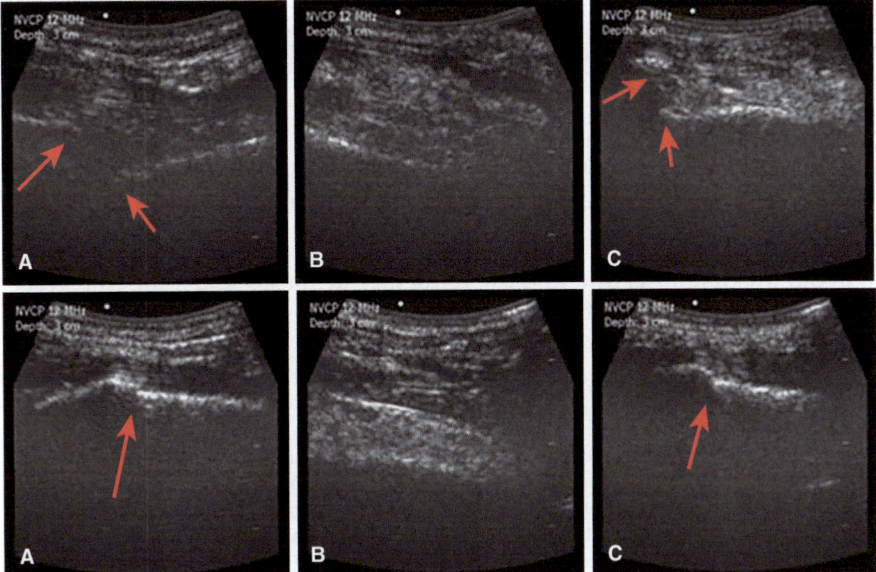

**Figure 22.8.** Distal radial fracture and postreduction assessment identifying disruption in cortical fracture lines identified by red arrows pre- and postreduction.

*Source*: From Lau, B. C., Robertson, A., Motamedi, D., & Lee, N. (2017). The validity and reliability of a pocket-sized ultrasound to diagnose distal radius fracture and assess quality of closed reduction. *The Journal of Hand Surgery*, 42 (6), 420–427. Used with permission from Elsevier, Inc.

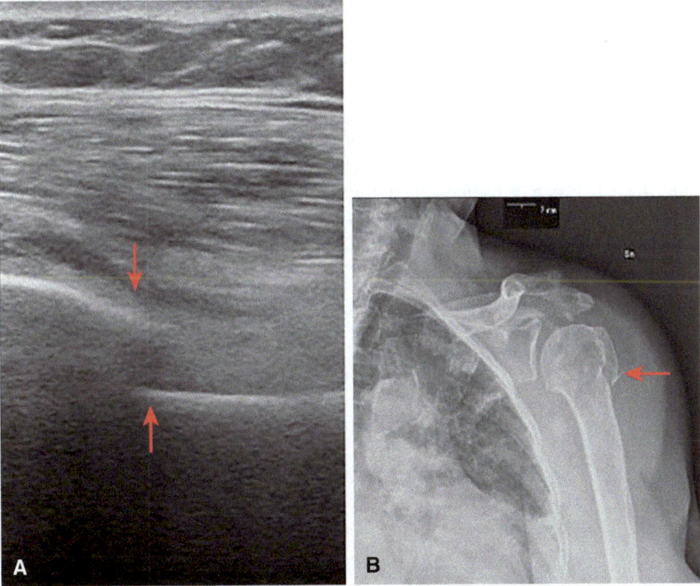

**Figure 22.9.** Ultrasound used to assess humerus fracture, compared to x-ray.

*Source*: From Caroselli, C., Zaccaria, E., Blaivas, M., Dib, G., Fiorentino, R., & Longo, D. (2020). A pilot prospective study to validate point of care ultrasound in comparison to X-ray examination in detecting fractures. *Ultrasound in Medicine & Biology*, 46(1), 11–19. https://doi.org/10.1016/j.ultrasmedbio.2019.09.006. Used with permission from Elsevier, Inc.

- Complex or comminuted fractures may be difficult to visualize via ultrasound.

- For complex fractures, complement the use of ultrasound with advanced imaging such as x-ray/CT/MRI.

- Difficult seeing subtle fractures.

- Engage in dynamic ultrasound; apply subtle pressure or ask pt to move the affected limb to better assess potentially nondisplaced fractures.

- Reverberation artifacts can mimic fractures.

- To avoid misdiagnosis due to these refractory artifacts, adjust the transducer angle and scan the bone from multiple planes. This will help differentiate a true fracture from artifact.

## BIBLIOGRAPHY

Champagne, N., Eadie, L., Regan, L., & Wilson, P. (2019). The effectiveness of ultrasound in the detection of fractures in adults with suspected upper or lower limb injury: A systematic review and subgroup meta-analysis. *BMC Emergency Medicine, 19*(1), 17. https://doi.org/10.1186/s12873-019-0226-5

Lau, B. C., Robertson, A., Motamedi, D., & Lee, N. (2017). The validity and reliability of a pocket-sized ultrasound to diagnose distal radius fracture and assess quality of closed reduction. *The Journal of Hand Surgery (American Ed.), 42*(6), 420–427. https://doi.org/10.1016/j.jhsa.2017.03.012

Leow, J. M., Clement, N. D., Tawonsawatruk, T., Simpson, C. J., & Simpson, A. H. R. W. (2016). The radiographic union scale in tibial (RUST) fractures: Reliability of the outcome measure at an independent centre. *Bone & Joint Research, 5*(4), 116–121. https://doi.org/10.1302/2046-3758 .54.2000628

Malik, H., Appelboam, A., & Nunns, M. (2021). Ultrasound-directed reduction of distal radius fractures in adults: A systematic review. *Emergency Medicine Journal, 38*(7), 537–542. https://doi.org/10.1136 /emermed-2020-210464

Nicholson, J. A., Tsang, S. T. J., MacGillivray, T. J., Perks, F., & Simpson, A. H. R. W. (2019). What is the role of ultrasound in fracture management? *Bone & Joint Research, 8*(7), 304–312. https://doi.org /10.1302/2046-3758.87.BJR-2018-0215.R2

Schmid, G. L., Lippmann, S., Unverzagt, S., Hofmann, C., Deutsch, T., & Frese, T. (2017). The investigation of suspected fracture—A comparison of ultrasound with conventional imaging. *Deutsches Ärzteblatt International, 114*(45), 757–764. https://doi.org/10.3238/arztebl.2017.0757

Wang, C. L., Shieh, J. Y., Wang, T. G., & Hsieh, F. J. (1999). Sonographic detection of occult fractures in the foot and ankle. *Journal of Clinical Ultrasound: JCU, 27*(8), 421–425. https://doi.org/10.1002/(sici) 1097-0096(199910)27:8<421::aid-jcu2>3.0.co;2-e

# CHAPTER 23

# SURGICAL AIRWAY

Ari Chaskes

## INTRODUCTION

- Percutaneous or surgical cricothyrotomy is a lifesaving procedure
- Setting: inability to ventilate or oxygenate in which nasal or orotracheal intubation is unable to be performed or unsuccessful
- Ultrasound aids in identifying upper airway anatomy, especially when landmarks are distorted due to trauma or edema.
- Ultrasound increases the successful identification of the cricothyroid membrane (CTM)
- Ultrasound measurements of upper airway anatomy augment difficult airway prediction
- Use of ultrasound to confirm endotracheal intubation demonstrates accuracy near 99.1% (Gottlieb et al., 2019)
- Ultrasound can improve first-pass success rates for surgical airways by identifying vascular structures and confirming tracheal location in real time.
- In the event there is no access to continuous capnography, ultrasound is an alternative per Advanced Cardiac Life Support (ACLS) guidelines (Gottlieb et al., 2019).

See Tables 23.1 and 23.2 for information on indications and differentials.

**Table 23.1** Indications

| Anticipation of difficult airway | Distorted anatomic landmarks | Trauma | Edema |
|---|---|---|---|
| Confirmation of ETT | Multiple intubation attempts | Obesity, short "bull" neck | Dyspnea, wheezing, cough, stridor |

ETT, endotracheal tube

**Table 23.2** Differentials

| Angioedema of face/tongue | Deep space neck infections (Ludwig angina, PTA) | Allergic reaction/anaphylaxis |
|---|---|---|
| Foreign body | Trauma | Epiglottitis |

PTA, peritonsillar abscess

## IMAGE ACQUISITION

- **Probe**
  - Linear

- **Preset**
  - Vascular
- **Hand placement**
  - Hold like a pencil
- **Technique**
  - Always maintain proper orientation
  - Scan in both the transverse and longitudinal planes
    - Transverse is usually quicker to view but not superior in accuracy
    - Longitudinal View "string of pearls technique," which can confirm proper midline placement.
      - Probe placed in the sagittal line from the thyroid cartilage to the caudal side
      - Cricothyroid membrane identified between cricoid and thyroid cartilage
    - Transverse view thyroid cartilage and cricoid cartilage air interface line (TACA)
      - Thyroid cartilage: Looks like triangular roof
      - Moving the probe caudally, the cricothyroid membrane appears as a bright hyperechoic line between the thyroid and cricoid cartilage.
      - Cricoid cartilage appears as a hypoechoic horseshoe structure shaped like black horseshoe
      - Cephalad to caudal: thyroid cartilage → air interface line → CTM → cricoid cartilage

## ANATOMY/IMAGES

See Figure 23.1 through Figure 23.2 for images depicting anatomy of the upper airway and cricothyroid membrane.

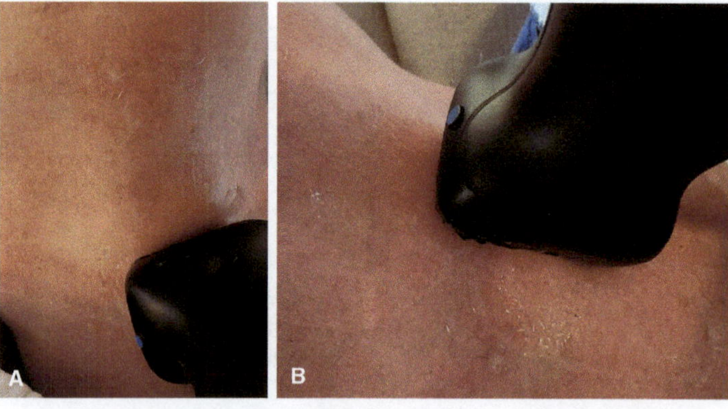

**Figure 23.1.** Anatomy of the upper airway. (A) Transverse plane. (B) Longitudinal plane.
*Source*: Used with permission. Image courtesy of Dr. Kelli Craven.

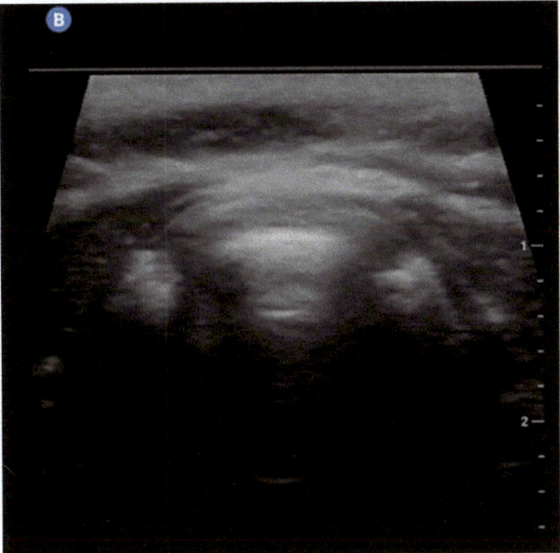

**Figure 23.2** Cricothyroid membrane with reverberation artifact. Transverse view.
*Source:* Used with permission. Image courtesy of Dr. Kelli Craven.

## INTERPRETATION

- Must visualize the cricothyroid membrane by identifying the hyperechoic air interface
- The cricothyroid membrane appears as a bright hyperechoic line between the thyroid and cricoid cartilage.
- Visualize the thyroid cartilage and cricoid cartilage
- The cricoid cartilage is the only complete cartilaginous ring of the airway and appears as a hypoechoic horseshoe structure on ultrasound.
- Visualize tracheal rings if scanning in a longitudinal axis

## PROCEDURE

- **Equipment**
  - Bougie and endotracheal tube (ETT)
  - Percutaneous cricothyrotomy kit
  - Antiseptic solution
  - 10 cc syringe
  - No. 11 blade scalpel
  - Tape
- **Patient/scanner position**
  - Patient
    - Supine with neck extended
  - Scanner
    - Right or left side of patient

- **Site selection**
  - Midsagittal plane over the neck
- **Procedure**
  - Ensure all equipment is available and proper patient position
  - Pre-load ETT onto bougie
  - Identify the cricothyroid membrane in both the longitudinal and transverse views
  - Once identified and the site is prepped, make a vertical incision through the skin over cricothyroid membrane
  - Make a horizontal incision through cricothyroid membrane, rotate the scalpel 90–180° to widen the opening, turning scalpel 180° to extend to both sides of the cartilaginous cage
  - Insert finger, blunt end of scalpel, or hemostat to pierce the membrane
  - Pass bougie alongside finger/scalpel/hemostat into trachea then remove
  - If resistance is met while advancing the bougie, slightly adjust the angle or twist the bougie to facilitate passage.
  - Pass endotracheal tube over bougie just until balloon disappears into trachea
  - Remove bougie and inflate the ETT cuff
  - Confirm placement with end-tidal $CO_2$ detector/colorimetric device
  - Ultrasound confirmation of endotracheal placement should show:
    - Single air-mucosal interface ("bullet sign") = correct tracheal intubation
    - Two air-mucosal interfaces ("double tract sign") = esophageal intubation
    - Confirm placement with US
  - Secure tube

**PRO TIP**

Utilize the US to verify lung sliding at second intercostal space bilaterally.

**PRO TIP**

NEVER let go of the ETT until secured.

- Obtain chest x-ray (CXR)

See Table 23.3 for a summary of pathologic findings.

**Table 23.3** Summary of Pathologic Findings

| Condition | Ultrasound Findings |
| --- | --- |
| Esophageal intubation | Observed "double tract" sign as the ETT is in the esophagus keeping it open lateral to the trachea in transverse view |
| Epiglottis | Larger and thickened epiglottis with epiglottitis |
| Vocal cord palsy or pathology | Visualized hypoechoic cyst structure or abnormal vocal cord movement |

*(continued)*

**Table 23.3** Summary of Pathologic Findings (*continued*)

| Condition | Ultrasound Findings |
| --- | --- |
| Tracheal location/displacement | Trachea does not sit midline when probe is in transverse axis over midline |
| Laryngeal injury | Soft tissue edema surrounding and discontinuity of thyroid cartilage |

ETT, endotracheal tube.

## PEARLS AND PITFALLS

- Use color Doppler to locate and avoid anterior jugular veins, which may cross over the cricothyroid membrane. Can use color flow Doppler to identify overlying vascular structures
- Ultrasound confirmation of endotracheal placement should show:
  - Single air-mucosal interface (bullet sign) = correct tracheal intubation
  - Two air-mucosal interfaces (double tract sign) = esophageal intubation
- Prediction of difficult laryngoscopy
  - Skin to epiglottis distance: >2.54 cm (sensitivity 82% and specificity 91%)
    - Predictor of difficult laryngoscopy
  - Hyomental distance ratio
    - Hyomental distance ratio of 1–1.05 in morbidly obese patients predicts difficult laryngoscopy
    - Hyomental distance ratio ranging 1.12–1.16 more easily intubated
- Hyomental distance ratio
  - Good indicator as a substitute of radiographic measurement of occipital-atlantoaxial joint extension (neck mobility which impacts difficult airway)
- US measurement of tongue base thickness to predict difficulty with mask ventilation
- Airway injury is 3 times more likely with digital palpation of airway landmarks without the use of POCUS.

**To access the videos, please go to the List of Videos in the front matter.**

## BIBLIOGRAPHY


Adi, O., Kok, M. S., & Wahab, S. F. A. (2019). Focused airway ultrasound: An armamentarium in future airway management. *Journal of Emergency and Critical Care Medicine, 3*(31), 1–10. https://jeccm.amegroups.org/article/view/5240/html

Favot, M. (2015). *Ultrasound for verification of endotracheal tube location.* Retrieved September 4, 2024, from https://www.aliem.com/ultrasound-for-verification-of-endotracheal-tube-location/

Gottlieb, M., Holladay, D., Nakitende, D., Hexom, B., Patel, U., Serici, A., Shah, S. C., & Bailitz, J. (2019). Variation in the accuracy of ultrasound for the detection of intubation by endotracheal tube size. *The American Journal of Emergency Medicine, 37*(4), 706–709. https://doi.org/10.1016/j.ajem.2018.07.026

Jain, K., Yadav, M., Gupta, N., Thulkar, S., & Bhatnagar, S. (2020). Ultrasonographic assessment of airway. *Journal of Anaesthesiology, Clinical Pharmacology, 36*(1), 5–12. https://doi.org/10.4103/joacp.JOACP_319_18

Lin, J., Bellinger, R., Shedd, A., Wolfshohl, J., Walker, J., Healy, J., Taylor, J., Chao, K., Yen, Y. H., Tzeng, C. T., & Chou, E. H. (2023). Point-of-care ultrasound in airway evaluation and management: A comprehensive review. *Diagnostics, 13*(9), 1541. https://doi.org/10.3390/diagnostics13091541

Nakazawa, H., Uzawa, K., Tokumine, J., Lefor, A. K., Motoyasu, A., & Yorozu, T. (2023). Airway ultrasound for patients anticipated to have a difficult airway: Perspective for personalized medicine. *World Journal of Clinical Cases, 11*(9), 1951–1962. https://doi.org/10.12998/wjcc.v11.i9.1951

Osman, A., & Sum, K. (2016). Role of upper airway ultrasound in airway management. *Journal of Intensive Care, 4*(1), 1–7. https://doi.org/10.1186/s40560-016-0174-z

Siddiqui, N., Arzola, C., Friedman, Z., Guerina, L., & You-Ten, K. E. (2015). Ultrasound improves cricothyrotomy success in cadavers with poorly defined neck anatomy: A randomized control trial. *Anesthesiology, 123*(5), 1033–1041. https://doi.org/10.1097/aln.0000000000000848